The Longevity Diet Recipes

This Book Includes: " Anti-inflammatory Diet Guide + The Affordable Air Fryer Cookbook"

By Tony Cook and Melissa William

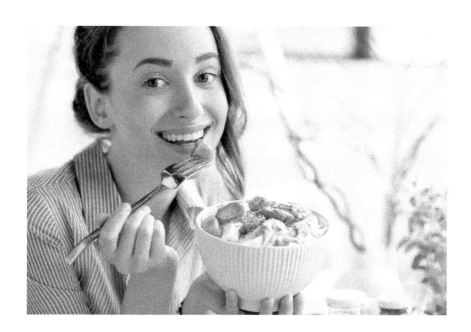

Legal & Disclaimer

The information contained in this book and its contents is not designed to replace or take the place of any form of medical or professional advice; and is not meant to replace the need for independent medical, financial, legal or other professional advice or services, as may be required. The content and information in this book has been provided for educational and entertainment purposes only.

The content and information contained in this book has been compiled from sources deemed reliable, and it is accurate to the best of the Author's knowledge, information and belief. However, the Author cannot guarantee its accuracy and validity and cannot be held liable for any errors and/or omissions. Further, changes are periodically made to this book as and when needed. Where appropriate and/or necessary, you must consult a professional (including but not limited to your doctor, attorney, financial advisor or such other professional advisor) before using any of the suggested remedies, techniques, or information in this book.

ANTI-INFLAMMATORY DIET GUIDE

THE AFFORDABLE AIR FRYER COOKBOOK

Anti-inflammatory diet guide

A comprehensive guide for the Anti-inflammatory diet plan, with healthy and tasty recipes to revitalize your life by losing weight and reducing long-term illness.

[Tony Cook]

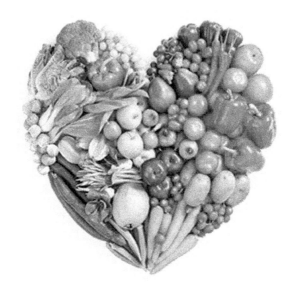

Legal & Disclaimer

The information contained in this book and its contents is not designed to replace or take the place of any form of medical or professional advice; and is not meant to replace the need for independent medical, financial, legal or other professional advice or services, as may be required. The content and information in this book has been provided for educational and entertainment purposes only.

The content and information contained in this book has been compiled from sources deemed reliable, and it is accurate to the best of the Author's knowledge, information and belief. However, the Author cannot guarantee its accuracy and validity and cannot be held liable for any errors and/or omissions. Further, changes are periodically made to this book as and when needed. Where appropriate and/or necessary, you must consult a professional (including but not limited to your doctor, attorney, financial advisor or such other professional advisor) before using any of the suggested remedies, techniques, or information in this book.

Upon using the contents and information contained in this book, you agree to hold harmless the Author from and against any damages, costs, and expenses, including any legal fees potentially resulting from the application of any of the information provided by this book. This disclaimer applies to any loss, damages or injury caused by the use and application, whether directly or indirectly, of any advice or information presented, whether for breach of contract, tort, negligence, personal injury, criminal intent, or under any other cause of action.

You agree to accept all risks of using the information presented inside this book.

You agree that by continuing to read this book, where appropriate and/or necessary, you shall consult a professional (including but not limited to your doctor, attorney, or financial advisor or such other advisor as needed) before using any of the suggested remedies, techniques, or information in this book.

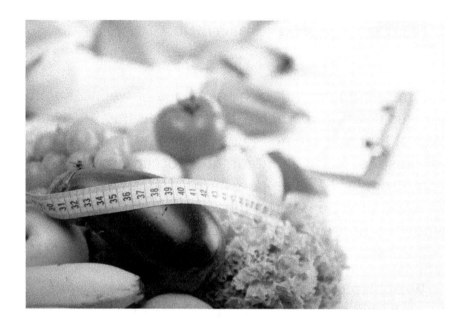

Book Description

Inflammation can hijack our feelings of wellness and slow us down, but when it becomes chronic, this may signal that something is out of alignment in our diet or lifestyle. Normal inflammation occurs in the body on a regular basis as part of our natural process of maintaining a healthy internal balance. It's only when the necessary process of inflammation gets out of hand that well-being can become impaired.

We'll also present the principles of an easy anti-inflammatory diet, based on whole foods and grounded in science, to support you in restoring your natural balance. Our simple lists of foods to include (and those to avoid) will help you choose meals far beyond the recipes. We'll also touch on how people's bodies respond differently to particular ingredients, so you can personalize these recipes to best meet your own nutritional needs.

The more difficult side of this equation is that the visceral fat is not one that ever truly leaves the body. It is the fat that hides out in all of the nooks and crannies of your abdominal organs, which makes it dangerous to remove with such invasive procedures as liposuction. Neither will these fat cells dissipate from your body with weight loss and exercise. However, as you reduce obesity levels, these fat cells respond by reducing in size, and that reduction slows down the production of as many harmful, inflammatory chemicals.

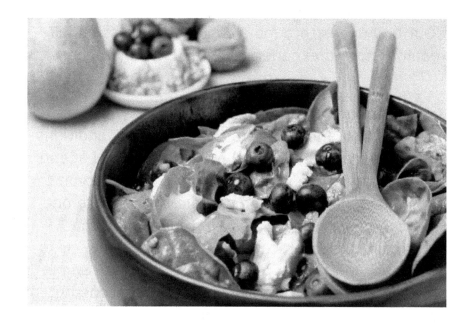

INTRODUCTION

A good and healthy diet can do miracles no medicine in this world can do. With a good diet, you can ensure a disease-free life with active metabolism. Our body goes through a constant process of self-repairment and experiences various phenomenon on the way.

Inflammations are therefore a temporary process of regeneration and reintegration of normal conditions following a damage; however, if the harmful agents persist or if there is a production of mainly type 1 cytokines, it can become chronic. In this case one can observe a progressive reduction of the microcirculation processes described above - as it happens during the recovery - while at the same time the infiltrated cells are progressively constituted by macrophages and lymphocytes that are frequently disposed around the vascular wall like a sleeve, which causes its compression. As a consequence, a state of tissue suffering is established, which is established by the presence of the infiltrate and by the reduction of blood flow caused by the vascular compression.

Inflammation is one of the body's responses to a number of environmental factors. The idea behind the conception of this book is to provide you with all the pros of opting a dietary approach to reduce or eliminate risks of inflammation and to make you aware of the relevant recipes. Let's get started!

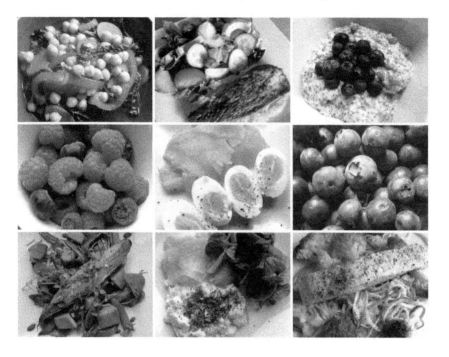

Chapter 1: What is Inflammation?

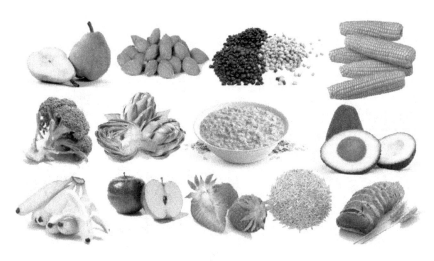

When using the terms inflammation or phlogosis one intends the set of alterations that occur in an area of the organism that has been hit by a damage of an intensity that has not affected the vitality of all cells within the area. Such damage could be induced by physical agents (such as traumas or heat), chemical agents (such as toxic components or acids) and biological agents (such as bacteria and viruses).

The response to the damage, the inflammation in fact, is given by the cells that have survived it and is therefore primarily a local reaction. Medical terminology defines the reaction by adding -tis to the name of the organ that is inflamed (for example the terms tendinitis and hepatitis indicate, respectively, a tendon and liver inflammation). The reaction was defined as primarily local instead of exclusively local as several molecules that are synthesized and released by the cells that participate in the phenomenon move into the blood and operate on long distanced organs, especially the liver. Thus, stimulating the liver cells to release other substances that are responsible for the acute response phase to the inflammation. The presence of a fever and leucorrhoea (which is an increase in the number of leukocytes circulating in the blood) represent other systematic indications of phlogosis. The inflammation itself is a useful process to the organism, as it allows it to neutralize (if present) the agent that has caused damage, and reintegrate the normal condition pre-existing to the detrimental event.

In the case of muscular injury, for example, the inflammation process that follows is especially necessary to activate a subdivided process of the very own damage (in this case the agent generating the damage would be a physical agent, like a trauma, and there will be no necessity to eliminate the damaging agent, unlike in other cases).

The most known symptoms of inflammations are an increase in the local temperature, swelling, redness, soreness, and functional compromission. The phenomenons that cause such symptoms are mainly caused by events that involve the microcirculation of blood. An extremely rapid vasoconstriction is followed by the relaxation of the smooth muscular fiber cells present on terminal arterioles' walls, with resulting vasodilation and increasing blood flow to the traumatized area (which causes the increase in local temperature and redness). Subsequently, the higher blood flow stagnates in the traumatized zone, thus increasing the blood's viscosity (given by the red blood cells' aggregation and by the plasma's outflow to the intercellular junctions); leukocytes will also start flowing out the blood at the extravascular compartment where they are attracted by specific cytokines. Thus, the exudate is formed, which is the root of the swelling. It is constituted partly by a liquid and partly by suspended cells in it. Finally, the subdivided process of cellular damage will start.

The set of processes that is described above is mediated by various molecules which trigger, maintain and also limit the modifications in the microcirculation. Such molecules are called chemical mediators of phlogosis, and they can come from different sources and have different scopes. These are histamine, serotonin, arachidonic acid's metabolites (prostaglandines, leukotrienes and thromboxanes), lysosomal enzymes, type 1 and type 2 cytokines, nitric oxide, the kinin system and the complement system. Instead, the cells that intervene in the inflammatory processes are constituted by mastocytes, basophils, neutrophils and eosinophils, monocytes/macrophages, natural killer cells, platelets, lymphocytes, plasma cells, endothelial cells and fibroblasts.

Next, fibroblasts can be stimulated to proliferate, with the consequence that many chronic phlogosis cases culminate with an excessive formation of connective tissue which constitutes fibrosis or sclerosis. For example, that is the case for cellulite, a socially unaesthetic disease which affects many women, caused by the increase in volume of adipose cells in some areas of the body (mostly thighs and glutes) with the lack of liquid draining and the process of local inflammation which can induce, at the worst phases, fibrosis and sclerosis with the formation of micronodules which give skin the classic "orange peel" aspect.

The inflammation itself can therefore be defined as a "physiologic" response of the organism to a detrimental stimulus (for example a cut or a trauma) and it can be of the acute kind (angio phlogosis), mainly involving the modifications to the vascular system to ease the reparation of the damage and the inflow of the immune system cells, or it can be chronic, of long duration and with a persistent reaction by the immune system. During these processes, it was clear how chemical mediators are generated in great quantities, such as inflammatory cytokines, which not only have a local action in the damaged tissue but also flow throughout the whole body and "inflame" it in chronic conditions.

That is the case, for example, for the pathological alterations of the Intestinal Microbiome (see related chapter) or more generally of the intestinal barrier with the diffusion of material from the enteric lumen in the blood flow and generation of a low level chronic inflammatory state.

Over time such conditions can increase the risk of many metabolic pathologies like obesity, diabetes mellitus and metabolic syndrome. Here is why it is good to know how to "deinflammate" our organism also through our diet choices.

Chapter 2: T of Inflammation?

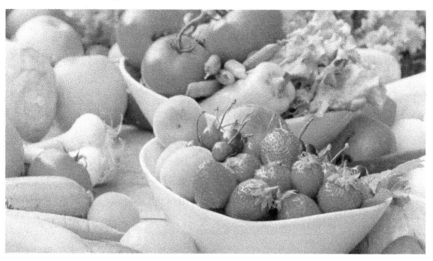

You should know the two major types of inflammation to better deal with it. These are:

Acute inflammation:

It is the instantaneous response of the body in the result of damage to body cells. Swelling occurs within 2 to 3 seconds of the injury. It doesn't persist for a longer duration.

Acute inflammation is one that starts quickly and becomes serious in a brief time. Signs or symptoms are normally just present for a couple of days and nights but may persist for a couple of weeks in some instances.

Systemic or Chronic inflammation:

It is a long-term inflammation, which is often caused due to allergies, cancer, diabetes, lungs diseases, asthma, heart complexities, etc. In these cases, the inflammation is cured only by treating the root cause.

Inflammation may be the defense reply that centers your immune system's consideration toward combating a perceived menace -- often microorganisms or Trojans or harm from international invaders, like poisons. When a section of your body becomes reddened, swollen, very hot and often agonizing, this is swelling in action.

Great up to now. But when swelling is chronically fired up, the immune system's capability to fight off different insects and pathogens will be compromised.

Chronic inflammation is frequently regarded as the effect of your "overactive" disease fighting capability -- as if your immune purpose is perplexed or malfunctioning. But can be this definitely what's going on? Or carry out we just reside in an increasingly harmful and stressful entire world?

After all, a lot of people today are confused with anxiety and environmental poisons, like endocrine-disrupting and cancer-causing substances from food to drinking water to household cleansers. And your body has every right to respond defensively. Foods allergies, poor diet program, toxins, and pressure are the most important culprits.

To combat irritation, we have to help our anatomies deal with this continuous harm of immune causes. One of the better ways to aid your body in combatting inflammation would be to consume an anti-inflammatory diet program.

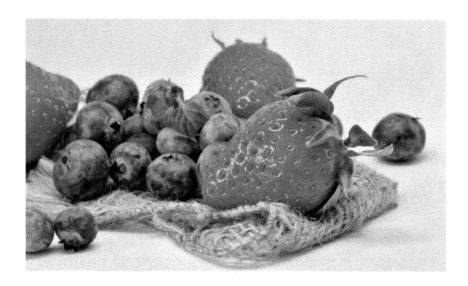

Chapter 3: Myths, misconceptions and mistakes made by individuals

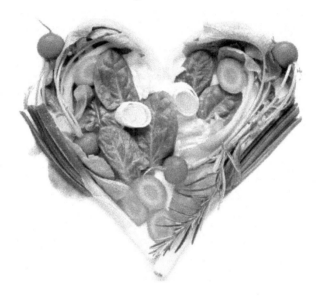

Your body's metabolism dictates your ability to produce energy. Metabolism is the process of breaking down food particles by the organic cells of your body. The metabolic process also plays a crucial role in your ability to burn fat to attain your ideal body weight.

Therefore, it is significant to your general health to have a high capacity of burning fat for energy. In short, it is always paramount to enhance your body's metabolic process.

Repeatedly, people are engaging in activities and behaviors. that are wrecking their metabolism.

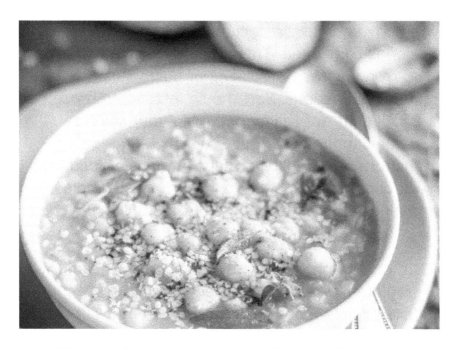

Worse, they are unaware of it all! The anti-inflammatory diet directly refers to the metabolic processes and the immune system of your body. Hence, therein gushes forth most of the common mistakes, misunderstandings, and misconceptions of practicing the regimen.

Here is a compilation of the top mistakes while practicing the regimen. Learning these common errors will help you to avoid these glitches along the way. The list also includes the corresponding tips:

Misstep #1: Concentrating on Calories & Heedless on Hormones

One of the most misinterpreted myths misguiding many people is the assumption that the weight of the body bears a direct connection to the number of calories consumed. This outdated perception is an erroneous way of looking at how your body's metabolic functions. You should instead embrace the significant reality of linking your caloric consumptions with your hormonal and body functions. The reality is that the types of food that you consume can alter your hormones completely and hinder the efficiency of your metabolism to burn fat.

In other words, consuming a calorically similar regimen of refined carbs against low-glycemic indexed whole foods will produce different effects on your metabolic processes. Likewise, indulging in a low-carb diet compared to a high-carb diet will cause advantageous outcomes on how your cells will burn fat for fuel, regardless of your caloric intake.

Again, your hormones and metabolism operate beyond food consumption. Your five primary hormones, which control your fat-burning process, are insulin, leptin, ghrelin, cortisol, and adiponectin. An array of factors influences these hormones such as your regular exercise routines, sleep quality, stress levels, hydration levels, and diet.

☐ Myth-1: Curb Carbs, Fill Fats

– Lowering your carb intakes and increasing your consumption of healthy fats makes a great difference towards improving your metabolism. Such a regimen simultaneously helps to stabilize your blood sugar levels, decreases insulin levels, and boosts the burning of fats. Consuming a surplus of carbs tends to convert the excesses into fats, stored as fatty tissues. Their regular consumption characterizes typically a chronically high blood sugar level, which results in a diverse range of destructive effects on your body.

However, switching your body into a fat-burning machine is technically engaging with a low-carb and high fat (LCHF) diet. Research supports this dietary model since it outperforms a low-fat regimen in countering obesity, diabetes, and other inflammatory factors.

☐ Myth-2: Short & Strenuous Exercise Engagements – Your exercise habits significantly contribute to the general health of your hormones.

Many people indulge in daily exercises with the aim of losing weight in the wrong way. Low-intensity cardio workouts daily are harmful to your body and as such, unnecessary.

Instead, short-duration and high-intensity intermittent exercises (HIIE) are highly effective for hormone enhancement. Modern studies confirm that these more explosive modes of exercises provide increased benefits for shedding weight as opposed to other forms of exercises.

Among the more well-known examples of these workouts are those boxing sessions or 30-second sprints followed by an active recovery activity of 2 to 4 minutes (usually, walking or other forms of low-intensity body movements). If ever you deem such exercises as severely intensive for your body, then you can always modify them.

An ideal phase, to begin with, would be 30 seconds of performing each exercise program, followed by another 30 seconds of resting. You may also Adjust the exercise movements to make them less straining or comfortably easier.

Nonetheless, your aim should be pushing yourself to your limits of performing high-intensity exercises. Attaining this objective allows your body to adapt to an appropriate hormonal balance gained from these typical exercises.

☐ Myth-3: Terminate Toxic Substances & Supplies – Accumulated toxins in your body can directly lead to poor fat metabolism. For instance, in today's modern society, many food chemical components can mimic the functions of estrogen (a hormone promoting fat retention) with potentials for completely disrupting a hormonal balance.

You can prevent exposing your body to such risks by eating only wild-caught or pasture-raised meats and organically grown vegetables. Furthermore, avoid using beauty products, synthetic plastics, unfiltered water, and other similar supplies filled with toxic substances.

Always be aware of what you introduce to your body. Check and use only products that contain natural ingredients as much as possible.

Misstep #2: Mindless on Micronutrients

For most of us, we spend the majority our time focusing more on our consumptions of fats, proteins, and carbohydrates— the major macronutrients. Although the amount of each of these macronutrients is a vital factor for healthy nutrition planning, the number of micronutrients may disputably be more significant. Your body uses dozens of various beneficial micronutrient substances.

These micronutrients include vitamins, minerals, fatty acids, enzymes, antioxidants, and all sorts of essential compounds contained in foods. Their role is to keep you energized, produce hormones and digestive enzymes, repair and rejuvenate cells and tissues, mineralize bones, slow down oxidation damage or aging caused by free radicals, and prevent nutritional deficiencies. Deficiencies of specific micronutrients may lead to various health issues such as bone loss, thyroid problems,poor digestion, and mental impairment. Notably, a low level of micronutrient consumption influences your body's metabolism directly in a manner that promotes a major gain of fats.

For instance, nutrients such as zinc, selenium, and iodine serve to produce thyroid hormones. When you severely lack these nutrients, you may incur lower thyroid hormone productions and a much slower metabolism.

☐ Myth-1: Rainbow Ration Regimen – Various colors in diverse foods represent the presence of corresponding types of nutrients and unique benefits. For instance:

☐ Red Foods – are rich in carotenoids that are beneficial for your heart, eyes, immune system, blood, joints, and skin.

☐ Orange Foods – are excellent sources of fiber and vitamin C that promote collagen growth. They also contain cryptoxanthins— antioxidants that protect cells from damage and cancer growths.

☐ Purple & Blue Foods – are high in powerful anthocyanins— antioxidants that protect against heart disease, improve mineral absorption, enhance exercise performance, boost brain function, and other highly anti-inflammatory mechanisms. Purple and blue foods can even synergize well with a high-fat regimen to accelerate fat burning.

☐ Green Foods – contain trace minerals, chlorophyll, and sets of the B-vitamins and Vitamin K that detoxify your body, fight free radicals, and improve your immune system.

In particular, green foods are leafy greens, which are ideal inclusions to low-carb nutrition that support fat metabolism.

☐ Yellow Foods – possess antioxidant compounds that convert into vitamins C, B6, and A, potassium, phosphorus, riboflavin, fiber, magnesium, and folate. All these help to improve your heart functions, vision, digestive, and immune systems.

☐ White Foods – have lots of vitamins, minerals, and other vital food nutrients that your body needs to maintain a healthy weight and to protect against various inflammatory diseases.

☐ Myth-2: Mineral Maintenance – Your body requires both major and minor trace minerals to maintain optimum wellness. These minerals are necessary for your enzymes to function appropriately apart from supporting essential metabolic processes such as thyroid hormone production.

Generally, the required amount of trace minerals for your body should be less than 100 milligrams a day.

The key trace elements are zinc, selenium, molybdenum, manganese, iron, iodine, copper, cobalt, and chromium.

They are nature's catalysts that stimulate the work of enzymes, which further generate all metabolic processes necessary for life.

Deficiencies in mineral intake disable your body to gain adequate energy, proper bone formation, blood circulation and maintain optimal levels of hormone production. Excellent sources of minerals include the following:

☐ Avocados

☐ Fermented Foods

☐ Ghee or Grass-Fed Butter

☐ Grass-Fed Meats

☐ Leafy Greens

☐ Olives

☐ Pasture-Raised Eggs

☐ Pink Salts

☐ Sea Vegetables

☐ Vegetable or Bone Broth

☐ Wild-Caught Fish

☐ Myth-3: Staple Supplements – Myopic or careless farming practices have resulted in poor soil conditions in several areas of the world. For this reason, it becomes more unreliable to determine whether farm products or the foods you eat contain proper levels of nutrients, which they should. Therefore, having a staple of daily food supplements is essential.

To cover all of your bases, an excellent strategy is to consume multi-vitamins, multi-minerals, or all-in-one superfoods. You do not necessarily need to take all these in one sitting, but consuming at least one of them is highly advisable, especially if you are nutrient-deficient.

A huge mistake most people commit is to leave their digestive problems unaddressed, particularly when trying to figure out their metabolism issues. Thus, if you are experiencing any digestive issues like leaky gut or dysbiosis (gut bacterial imbalance), reduced stomach acids, and small intestinal bacterial overgrowth (SIBO), then it is difficult for your body to regulate hunger, much less, absorb all the food nutrients.

Furthermore, your body will have a sluggish metabolism that will leave you overweight and feeling lethargic. Poor digestion may also cause an undesirable spiral of effects that stifle your metabolism and thyroid hormone conversion.

Misstep #3: Availing Needlessly Anti-Nutrients

Anti-nutrients either deplete or prevent absorption of other useful nutrients in your body. They may manifest in various forms such as the following:

☐ Toxins – heighten the demand for detoxifying the liver. The delicate detoxification process requires the involvement of various multiple nutrients. These nutrients somehow include food products that contain antibiotics, artificial sweeteners, heavy metals,herbicides, pesticides, and other chemical elements within or on them.

The most common types of these toxic anti-nutrients are non-organic foods and processed vegetable oils. Both food items highly tend to contain pesticides, which damage your gut and deplete nutrients from your body.

Processed vegetable oils do not provide your body with a source of fuel. Besides, they are highly inflammatory. The more you consume them, the more you should eat consume omega-3 fats just to offset the harmful effects.

☐ Sugars –stimulate the process of glycolysis (breaking down sugars and carbohydrates), thus causing high sugar levels in the blood. These processes deplete vitamins B, C, and D, as well as calcium, chromium, and magnesium minerals in your body.

When consumed in excess, sugars may even lead to disruptions in cellular energy production. In effect, energy deficiencies slow down the protective mechanisms of metabolism.

☐ Phytates, Lectins, and Oxalates – are plant-based anti-nutrient proteins and compounds. People are often unaware of eating them because they are essential constituents of many everyday food items.

Plants are immobile and unable to protect themselves from various predators by either a 'fight or flight' response. Instead, they create compounds— phytates, lectins, and oxalates— that are micro toxins or poisonous for their predators.

☐ Myth-1: Avoid Anti-Nutrients Necessarily – Limiting your intakes of anti-nutrients requires you to know their chief origins. For instance, phytates generally come from legumes, grains, and nuts. While phytates are healthy for your body, they constrict the absorption of minerals such as zinc, magnesium, and calcium. Oxalates are commonly present in beets, cacao, nuts, raspberries, seeds, and spinach. Lectins are predominant in nightshade vegetables, seeds, nuts, legumes, and grains.

You do not need to avoid them altogether, but it is prudent to lessen your consumptions of these plant-based anti-nutrients. Otherwise, you will eventually incur serious gut health issues, chronic pain, or kidney problems.

☐ Myth-2: Soaking & Steaming Preparation Procedures – To further augment the reduction of anti-nutrient content in some foods, you should practice soaking seeds and nuts in filtered water right on the eve before you use or consume them. Some nuts and seeds may sprout after soaking them. These processes of soaking and sprouting unveil a higher nutritional profile, making the nuts and seeds more suitable for your digestive tract.

Raw cruciferous (mustard family) of vegetables can be direct sources of anti-nutrients, which pose difficulties on your digestive tract. A better way to lessen the disabling effects of these typical vegetables is to steam them before eating. Steaming also serves to break down exterior cellulose fibers gently, and thus, making it easier for your digestive tract system to process. Fermenting is also another viable option.

Misstep #4: Treating Thirst as Hydrating Hunger

Mostly, people easily misinterpret thirst for hunger. Yet the reality is that a dehydrated body can convey a false signal to your brain, indicating a low blood sugar and prompt you to eat.

If you are engaging in a low-carb dietary plan and frequently end up feeling hungry between meals, then, you are either dehydrated or not eating enough fats. Hence, instead of grabbing immediately for a snack, drink a glass of water first and observe how you feel.

☐ Myth-1: Win Wellness with Water – Hydration is crucial on any dietary program. However, there are several recommendations for adequate water intake.

Studies note that all it takes to impair your physical performances is a water loss equivalent to 2% of your body weight. A water loss of roughly 2.8% of your body weight can reduce your cognitive functions. By these conclusions, it is vital to reiterate how your ideal water intake directly relates to your body weight.

As a basic guideline, your daily minimum water intake should be half of your total body weight (based in pounds) in ounces of water. Ideally, you should consume ¾ of your entire body weight in ounces of water per day. This recommendation is highly unlikely if you weigh more than 3,000 pounds. Nevertheless, if you are slim and lean, this advice is simple to follow as long as you stay hydrated between meals.

Applying baseline values, consider drinking more to refill the water lost from exercising. The same studies suggest that for water lost due to exercises, you should drink a half-liter (18-ounces) of water for each pound of your total body weight.

Hence, drinking water amidst your diet demands you to weigh yourself daily. This procedure allows you to know how much weight you have already lost or what weight you should ideally maintain.

Nonetheless, one of the more popular hydration strategies is to hydrate your body early in the day. For instance, drinking 1-2 liters (16-32 ounces) of water before taking your first meal is an excellent way of cleansing the body, promoting better digestion, and restoring dehydration that has just occurred overnight.

In addition, proper hydration of your body is dependent on both water and mineral contents. Combining a pinch of sea salt with your water is a bright idea to add electrolytes— body minerals found in the bloodstream, tissues, urine, and other body fluids that help to balance water retention in your body

Adding organic acids (i.e., citric and acetic acids) in your water is also a great way to improve your body's hydration and stabilize your blood sugar level. You can consume these acids in the form of lemon juice (citric acid) or apple cider vinegar (acetic acid). You only have to add a splash of either organic acids to your water to curtail your cravings until mealtime.

Chapter 4: How Dieting works

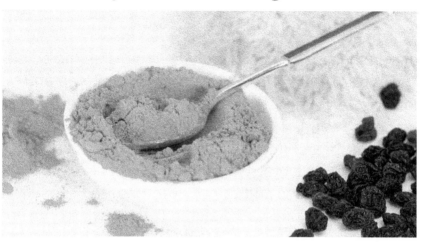

Inflammation has always been a therapeutic secret, yet now it has turned into a foe of long haul health. Additional red platelets, safe cells, and antioxidants are hurrying to the injured site to recuperate it. In any case, conveyed excessively thus far,inflammation can be lethal, as when somebody is too scorched to even consider recovering.

Just in a couple that is previous of, has it unfolded that low-level incessant inflammation, which ordinarily goes unnoticed, has an influence on numerous life disorders, for example, hypertension, heart disease, cancer, and Alzheimer's disease.

The moderate trickle, dribble of inflammatory markers, can take a very long time to make real impedance, which implies that every individual must tailor his way of life to counter them. Diet alone is not sufficient to keep ceaseless, intense inflammation under control... yet it is a decent start. The Mediterranean diet has been known to help lessen inflammation in the body, so it is an incredible way to kick-start your diet. By embracing an anti-inflammatory diet, you go for two positive outcomes: keeping the microorganisms in your digestive tracts healthy and flourishing, thereby avoiding the drainage of lethal synthetics into the circulation system. There is additionally the circuitous benefit that a healthy stomach related framework, sends a sign of prosperity along the vagus nerve to the heart and cerebrum. There is a huge number of microorganisms that possess the intestinal tract, and are a fundamental piece of our complete DNA, contributing a great many separate genomes. Together this tremendous settlement is known as the microbiome. Here are some basic focuses to know. The gut microbiome is not the same as a culture to culture.

In every one of us, it is always moves accordingly to the diet, yet to pressure and even feelings. Because of its hereditary, multifaceted nature, an "ordinary" gut microbiome has not been characterized at this point. It is accepted that flourishing, healthy gut microbiome is

established on a wide scope of common foods wealthy in fruits, vegetables, and fiber. The cutting edge Western diet, which is low in fiber, yet high in sugar, salt, fat, and handling food, might be genuinely debasing the gut microbiome. At the point when the gut microbiome is harmed or debased, microscopic organisms start to discharge supposed endotoxins— the results of microbial activity. If these poisons spill through the intestinal divider into the circulatory system, markers for inflammation are activated, and persevere until the poisons are never again present.

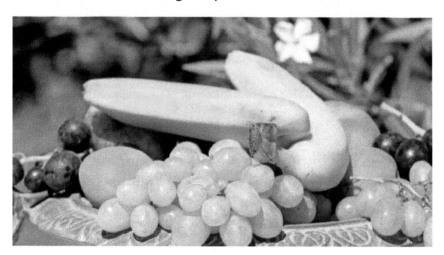

Chapter 5: An overview of Anti-Inflammatory Diet

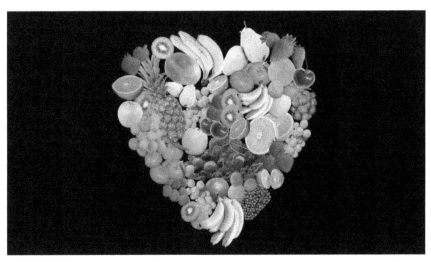

How Inflammation Helps—and Harms

When the immune system is working properly, inflammation plays an important role in our body's healthy response to injury or infection. Upon injury or infection, such as a scrape on the knee or exposure to the cold everyone else has at the office, our immune system rallies to restore health. This leads to a period of acute inflammation, which promotes healing as the body's defensive process repairs and restores integrity. Once the problem has been successfully managed, the immune response deactivates, and the inflammation around the area of injury or infection subsides.

When you notice that a paper cut on your finger is red, swollen, warm, and painful, this is all part of inflammation, which is taking place as a result of a smoothly running immune system. Immune cells have been activated to the site of the problem, so blood flow in the area increases, leading to the experience of swelling and heat, which will subside as the wound heals. Soon you'll have nothing to remember the paper cut by but a thin line of scar tissue. This kind of acute, localized inflammation may not require any additional treatment; however, maintaining a consistent anti-inflammatory diet like the one described in this book will ensure that your body has all the nutrients needed to support even this minor healing process.

Conversely, a little cut that seems to hang on too long, remaining puffy and painful and not making much progress in healing, might indicate a bigger issue. In this case, the normal process of acute inflammation may have continued unchecked, signaling a chronic inflammation that is more problematic. This can occur as a result of an unhealed infection like hepatitis B or C, prolonged exposure to environmental toxins like cigarette smoke, or existing health conditions like obesity or autoimmune disease. Lifestyle factors such as diet and stress can also amplify the inflammatory response. At first, there may not be any obvious symptoms of this kind of ongoing low-grade inflammation, yet in the long term, chronic inflammation can increase risk for or exacerbate a variety of diseases.

ANTI-INFLAMMATORY DIET GUIDELINES

Smart Dietary Choices

A whole foods approach to eating is the best route to decreasing inflammation, and that's the strategy we present here. As the benefits of anti-inflammatory diets become clearer, a growing number of studies reveal which foods are best to include or avoid as you move toward vibrant wellness. Let's check them out.

Foods That Fight Inflammation

FRUITS AND VEGETABLES. Consider yourself free to enjoy a wide range of fruits and vegetables on the anti-inflammatory diet—they're all good! Plant foods deliver a high-nutrient, low-calorie foundation and add bright, tempting color to any plate. These foods are a source of satisfying, anti-inflammatory fiber, plus vitamins, minerals, and micronutrients. Fruits and vegetables also contain powerful antioxidant compounds that help prevent cellular damage.

Berries, watermelon, apples, and pineapple in particular are proven anti-inflammatory superstars, thanks to their high levels of phytonutrients. Thousands of these chemicals can be found in different combinations in plant foods, and while they protect the plant against environmental damage, they also protect you on a cellular level, especially when you eat a wide range of produce. Citrus fruits provide high-antioxidant vitamin C, a knockout inflammation fighter. Vegetables such as onions, broccoli, and leafy greens support resistance to inflammation. Garlic and onion don't just add pungent flavor—they've also been studied extensively for their immune system benefits.

NIGHTSHADES. Beware the boundless Internet (mis)information available—some is inaccurate and not well grounded in science. Rumors that you can't enjoy nightshades such as tomatoes, potatoes, bell peppers, and eggplant on an anti-inflammatory diet are unfounded for most people. While some with autoimmune conditions like rheumatoid arthritis choose to avoid these nutritious vegetables, the Arthritis Foundation notes that no scientific data supports this, and in fact, the group cites research that shows that consumption of yellow and purple potatoes may actually lower inflammation. However, you are the expert of your own body. If you find that this restriction is supportive of your own health and well-being, then just try to include a wide range of other vegetables to ensure you are providing all the nutrition your body needs to heal. For most people, nightshade vegetables are part of a nutritious, anti-inflammatory diet. For instance, compounds such as the lycopene provided by cooked tomatoes make these vegetables standouts for fighting inflammation.

WHOLE AND ANCIENT GRAINS. Whole and ancient grains don't merely replace refined grains. They provide exciting flavors and textures, along with fiber, micronutrients, antioxidants, and protein. Naturally gluten-free grains, such as quinoa and amaranth, keep meals interesting and can be enjoyed by everyone.

GOOD FATS. We have learned that it's more important to enjoy the right kinds of fats in moderation than to try to eliminate fat altogether. Olive oil is a rich source of polyphenols, which are compounds shown to reduce indicators of inflammation, and it should be your primary cooking oil. Specialty oils like walnut oil or pumpkin seed oil add rich flavor and beneficial unsaturated fats. And we're happy to promote the benefits of dark chocolate, a delicious source of protective polyphenols—and a fine end to a meal!

OMEGA-3 FATTY ACIDS ARE ALL-STAR ANTI-INFLAMMATORY FATS. Include foods with this type of unsaturated fat frequently to optimize your whole diet approach. Fatty fish like salmon and sardines are excellent sources, as are some plant foods such as walnuts and flaxseed. Flaxseed may sound foreign, but it's been around for thousands of years, just now gaining popularity for its abundant fiber, protein, and powerful antioxidants called lignans. Consumption of flaxseed protects against inflammation and some cancers, but go for the ground version, so your body can absorb all that goodness. Seeds like hemp and chia are similarly helpful, as are pine nuts, which are actually nutrient-dense seeds.

HERBS AND SPICES. With countless options, each herb and spice has a unique profile of antioxidants and bright flavors to complement all kinds of cuisine. Turmeric deserves special mention for its proven anti-inflammatory and neuroprotective properties. Ginger, saffron, and cinnamon are other potent flavor enhancers worth trying. Herbs such as basil, rosemary, and thyme all have inflammation-fighting compounds, and their aroma and taste elevate the meal experience.

PROBIOTICS AND PREBIOTICS. What are these, anyway? Probiotics and prebiotics support immune and digestive health. Fermented foods such as yogurt, sauerkraut, pickles, tempeh, and kimchi are known as probiotic foods because they provide a direct infusion of healthy bacteria to your system in addition to their characteristic tang. Prebiotics are foods that feed those good gut bacteria—sources include high-fiber vegetables, whole grains, and beans. Cooked beans like black beans, chickpeas, and lentils also double as lean, plant-based proteins.

HEALTHY DRINKS. Washing foods down with kombucha keeps the probiotic theme going, although not everyone appreciates the sour taste of this fermented beverage! Thankfully, unsweetened teas are good beverage options—green tea is a particularly robust source of antioxidants. Drip coffee provides fiber and is one of the biggest contributors of antioxidants to the American diet—just try to keep it sugar-free. A glass of red wine from time to time provides protective resveratrol. Water is always a great choice for hydration and promotes the body's ability to detoxify at the cellular level.

OWN YOUR WATER

Water can be the most refreshing treat when you're parched. A decanter of water with sliced cucumber in a hotel lobby is a welcome sight to weary travelers. Yet it's amazing to see how many people have a hard time taking in enough water each day. If you're one of them, consider adding some fruits or herbs to your water to boost the flavor and the benefits. Buy a pretty glass pitcher; it will make the water look especially inviting. Ginger, thyme, basil, and rosemary make good herbal anti-inflammatory add-ins; beneficial fruits include orange, grapefruit, lemon, lime, apples, watermelon, and pineapple. Try water infused with blueberries and lemon, cucumber and mint, or beets and rosemary—or come up with your own favorite flavor combinations!

Foods That Worsen Inflammation

PROCESSED FOODS. There is no shortage of delicious, nourishing food to enjoy on your anti-inflammatory diet. To maximize the benefits, you'll want to leave behind those highly processed, packaged foods, as they are typically full of proinflammatory sodium, saturated fats, added sugars, and refined grains such as white flour or white rice.

AVOID ADDED SUGARS AND REFINED GRAINS FROM ANY SOURCE. These proinflammatory foods dramatically increase blood sugar, have more calories than they do nutrition, and are linked to many negative health effects.

PROCESSED AND RED MEAT. Some meats, such as ham and many deli meats, are highly processed and contain undesirable saturated fat and sodium. Red meat is another food to choose less frequently. Even lean cuts are likely to have high levels of proinflammatory saturated fats. You might be surprised to know that you should save backyard cookouts for special occasions. This is because fatty proteins like beef prepared with high-heat dry cooking methods increase production of proinflammatory substances called advanced glycation end products, or AGEs. Consider using lower-heat, moist cooking methods, such as stewing, sautéing, or poaching, to minimize this effect. Select lean, grass-fed beef options that offer protective omega-3s, in contrast with regular beef, which is high in proinflammatory omega-6 fats.

Foods to Consider with Care

Many foods fall in the middle of the health spectrum—these foods are neither the foundation of an anti-inflammatory diet nor the worst choices. These should be considered with care, depending on your own goals and current health condition. These foods are used sparingly in our recipes, and when we do include them, we offer substitutions.

CERTAIN OILS. A few plant-based oils should be approached thoughtfully. Corn, safflower, sunflower, and soy oils are high in proinflammatory omega-6s. Despite the trendiness of coconut oil on websites that promise "magic results" from consuming it in high amounts, it is a highly saturated fat, and there is no reason to believe it is healthy to consume in excess. Occasional dishes can be prepared with coconut oil, but keep olive oil as your go-to kitchen staple.

SKIN-ON DARK-MEAT POULTRY AND PORK. Skinless white-meat poultry can serve as a good source of protein. However, higher-fat dark meat and poultry with skin-on are less healthful. Many pork products contain too much fat and sodium to belong in an anti-inflammatory diet, but very lean pork, such as pork tenderloin, can be enjoyed occasionally.

NATURAL SUGARS. We all deserve a treat, and nobody wants to feel deprived. When your sweet tooth does strike, the best sweets to choose, in moderation, are natural sugars such as honey, maple syrup, and molasses rather than refined sugar products. These offer some trace micronutrients, along with the sweet taste we crave.

Unique Bodies, Unique Reactions to Food

We also treat the "Big 8" food allergens (fish, shellfish, peanuts, tree nuts, wheat, soy, eggs, and dairy) as "Consider with Care" foods, to highlight them for those individuals who need to make substitutions. Food allergies are immune system responses in which the body mistakenly responds to proteins, in otherwise wholesome foods, as a threat. Food allergies can be life threatening, and those with food allergies know they must be vigilant to ensure they are not accidentally consuming foods that will stimulate a negative immune response.

Some people have sensitivities and intolerances to particular foods that are not technically allergies, as they do not involve the immune system. The research into this area is growing but still inconclusive; for many individuals, the best barometer for food tolerance comes from simply paying attention to how you feel after consuming that food. You know your own body best, so please modify the diet we present here to your needs. If you are uncertain about how well a particular food fits into your own dietary pattern, keep note of how you react when you eat that food, and consider consulting with a registered dietitian.

For those who can consume fish and shellfish, these are potent inflammation fighters. Deep-water fish offer unparalleled amounts of omega-3 fats in a form that is very easy for the body to use in fighting inflammation, so salmon and herring can be regular staples of your diet if you are not allergic.

Peanuts and tree nuts (walnuts, cashews, etc.) are anti-inflammatory powerhouses. If you're able to eat them, small portions of almonds or pecans provide the antioxidant vitamin E, healthy fats, and a bit of protein in addition to their rich, satisfying crunch.

Most people can consume nutritious ancient grains with no problems. If you have celiac disease or are intolerant or allergic to gluten, you'll want to avoid wheat berries and barley. Ancient grains may be avoided on strict elimination diets, which are not necessary for most people wanting to reduce inflammation. We also list the more processed whole-grain products under "Consider with Care." Whole-wheat bread is a step in the right direction from white bread, but it is still highly processed.

Intact whole grains such as quinoa reign supreme for their anti-inflammatory power.

Soy is a major allergen but also a powerful inflammation fighter. Despite widespread myths, research shows that soy reduces inflammation and cancer risks for most people—great news if you enjoy popping steamed edamame in your mouth at your favorite sushi restaurant! Soy is a high-protein source of fiber, so unless you have an allergy, freely include edamame and tofu in your diet.

Eggs offer micronutrients such as choline and lutein, but they're another common allergen. While they do not appear to have specifically anti-inflammatory properties, they can serve as a good protein source in a healthy, balanced diet. If you can, consider including eggs as part of your overall dietary strategy.

Dairy is another major food allergen. Low- or non-fat dairy products, and those cultured to provide probiotics, like yogurt and kefir, should be considered with care. There is controversy over the benefits of including full-fat dairy in one's diet, but in relation to inflammation, the picture is clearer. Sources of saturated fat, like butter and cream, are best limited on an anti-inflammatory diet, so we don't use them here.

Anti-Inflammatory Food Lists

Foods in the "Enjoy" section can be eaten freely by most people. Challenge yourself to try them all! "Consider with Care" foods are nutritious for many people to consume as part of an otherwise balanced meal pattern. If you have a food allergy or other health consideration, choose one of the other options provided. The "Avoid" foods promote inflammation and can derail your efforts. Look for ways to swap those out for foods on the "Enjoy" list!

Benefits You'll See

Change can be hard—even positive change! As you begin this diet, you may find yourself challenged as you begin thinking about your meal choices in unfamiliar ways. That's a great reason to use the shopping lists and meal plans as we've presented them. This will take the guesswork and decision making out of the early stages of your transition to an anti-inflammatory lifestyle. Then you'll build confidence to begin testing out variations that work for you.

At first, you will notice that you are satisfied after each meal or snack, and that the energy you feel is more lasting throughout your day. You may find yourself getting hungry less often; this is because you're consuming more nutrient-dense foods. You may even see your skin clearing up as you remove highly processed foods and added sugars and replace them with more nourishing options that support health at the cellular level. Many people who shift to this eating style report gradual weight loss over time, which is also beneficial for reducing inflammation.

Less visible but equally important are the longer-term improvements you may notice in your health. If you happen to get a blood test from your doctor, you'll probably see the markers of inflammation, such as C-reactive protein (CRP) and interleukin 6 (IL-6), going down, and a more healthy lipid profile—higher HDL ("good") cholesterol and lower LDL ("bad") cholesterol—emerging over time. Your energy will likely be increasingly vibrant yet grounded and calm, and your body will be better able to fight off infection, whether that means just a little cold or a more significant threat. Your energy will increase, you will be better equipped to manage stress, and you'll just feel better—all qualities that can't be quantified in a lab test. Rather, you'll notice it when you bound out of bed in the morning, feeling great and ready to tackle the day—after a nourishing and satisfying anti-inflammatory breakfast, that is!

FOODS TO ENJOY

VEGETABLES (FRESH, FROZEN, OR CANNED WITHOUT ADDED SODIUM)

Alliums

Chives

Garlic*

Leeks

Onions*

Scallions

Shallots

Cruciferous Vegetables*

Arugula

Bok choy

Broccoli

Brussels sprouts

Cabbage

Cauliflower

Collard greens

Kale

Kohlrabi

Mizuna

Mustard greens

Radish greens

Romanesco broccoli/Roman cauliflower

Turnip greens

Dark Green Leafy Vegetables

Lettuces, especially romaine*

Spinach*

Swiss chard*

Root Vegetables

Beets

Carrots

Celery root/celeriac

Radishes

Rutabagas

Sweet potatoes

Turnips

Winter squash

Other Vegetables

Asparagus

Bell peppers

Corn

Fermented, probiotic vegetables*

Green beans

Mushrooms

FRUIT (FRESH, FROZEN, OR CANNED WITHOUT ADDED SUGAR)

Apples

Apricots

Avocados

Bananas

Berries*

Citrus*

Cranberries

Figs

Grapes

Kiwi

Mangos

Melons

Pineapple*

Stone fruit

FATS AND OILS

Nut oils

Olive oil*

Seed oils

WHOLE AND ANCIENT GRAINS

Amaranth*

Brown rice

Buckwheat*

Millet*

Oatmeal*

Popcorn

Quinoa*

Teff*

SEEDS

Chia

Flaxseed*

Hemp

Mustard

Poppy

Pumpkin

Sesame

Sunflower

HERBS AND SPICES

Basil

Bay leaf

Cilantro

Cinnamon*

Clove

Dill

Ginger*

Mint

Nutmeg

Oregano*

Paprika

Parsley

Pepper

Rosemary*

Saffron*

Sage

Tarragon

Thyme

Turmeric*

PROTEINS

Beans*

Tempeh*

Tofu

OTHER

Unsweetened coffee

Unsweetened black or green tea*

Note: Asterisks indicate foods that are particularly beneficial anti-inflammatory superstars.

CONSIDER WITH CARE

FATS AND OILS

Coconut

Corn

Safflower

Sesame

Soy

Sunflower

WHOLE AND ANCIENT GRAINS

Barley

Emmer

Farro

Rye

Spelt

Wheat berries

Whole-grain breads, bulgur, couscous, pastas

NUTS AND SEEDS

Peanuts

Tree nuts* (e.g., almonds, cashews, macadamias, pistachios, walnuts*)

DAIRY

Fermented, probiotic dairy* (e.g., kefir, yogurt)

Low-fat and non-fat dairy products (e.g., cheese, milk)

PROTEINS

Eggs

Fish* (e.g., cod, flounder, halibut, mackerel, salmon,* sardines,* tuna)

Pork (very lean cuts, such as pork tenderloin)

Poultry (skinless white meat)

Shellfish (e.g., mussels, oysters, scallops)

Soy (e.g., edamame/soybeans, tofu, tempeh)

OTHER

Dark chocolate

Red wine

AVOID

FATS AND OILS

Butter

Lard

Margarine

GRAINS

All refined grains (e.g., white bread and rolls, white pasta, white rice)

Packaged, processed grain-based snacks and desserts (e.g., biscuits, cakes, cereals, cookies, crackers, muffins)

Pastries

OTHER

Bacon

Beef (especially high-fat cuts, beef charred on the grill, and corn-fed beef—typically any that is not grass-fed)

Full-fat dairy (e.g., butter, cheese, cream, half-and-half, ice cream)

High-fat foods (especially those with high saturated fats or trans fats)

High-sodium foods

Packaged and processed foods

Packaged, processed meat alternatives (e.g., "garden burgers," faux chicken)

Refined added sugars (brown sugar, confectioners' sugar, high-fructose corn syrup, white sugar)

Chapter 6: Weight Loss and the Importance of Calories

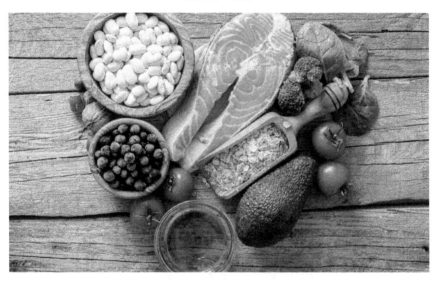

Obesity is one of these, especially if you have one of those "apple-shaped" body types where you are thicker around the middle. As previously noted, the visceral belly fat that hangs out among the organs of your abdomen does produce more of the markers in your blood stream that tell your physician that you are suffering from inflammation. The more of this "belly fat" that can be reduced, the better control you have over the reduction of those produced chemicals that aid in the development and flare ups of inflammation.

<u>Lose Weight and Feel Great with the Anti-Inflammatory Diet</u>

By slimming down, diminishing the amount of body fat you hold all together, you will begin to decrease the size of those visceral fat cells. The nice, added benefits include a weight loss that helps decrease or eliminate extra pressure on our joints and organs, in turn helping to alleviate some of the pain initially compounded by the inflammation.

One example that helps to explain this is the ratio of pounds to pressure on the knees. One extra pound of weight on your body exerts four extra pounds of pressure on your knees. It is how the body is built to distribute the weight. This means that by losing only ten pounds, you will reduce the amount of pressure on your knees by forty pounds!

Consider how it feels lifting forty pounds of groceries from the car (there are many who can't even do that much in one shot). Think about how you feel when you carry them into the house. The movement, the walking, etc. Adds that additional pressure to the joints of the knees, not to mention the arms, shoulders, and back. When they are put down, your body heaves a little sigh of relief. That extra weight pulling and pressing on our joints and muscles can hurt!

When you lose ten pounds, you are removing an extra forty pounds in just pain and pressure on the knees, let alone how it affects your other joints and muscles. Your body becomes more agreeable and maybe nags you just a little less. After all, pain is the body's way of telling you that something needs to change. It is protecting itself. You are coming to an agreement with your body that you will stop and reduce the pressure that you have been putting on it, while it, in turn, responds by agreeing to reduce the pain it has been causing with its nagging for you to take better care of it.

Let's take a look at a few other things that can help you have more agreeable communication with your body. Movement is one of these. If you are like most people, when you are in pain, or even feeling the general "ick" that comes with inflammation, the last thing you feel like is moving or doing anything that will draw your attention to the pain. And yet, what happens when you sit too long in one position and then have to get up and move anyway, for whatever reason? Your muscles and joints groan loudly in protest because they were quite comfortable with sitting still, pretending they didn't hurt in the first place. Your immediate reaction is usually one of not wanting to move because it hurts, and no one wants to hurt!

But we all do have to move at some point. When you start from a place of inaction—non-movement—your muscles and connective tissues for the joints stubbornly tighten up. It takes you a moment or more to get moving again, as you have to push past the tightness, which admittedly tends to hurt more at the beginning and then usually lessens as you keep going. By making movement a natural part of your day, you reduce the amount of stiffness that sets in, in turn reducing the amount of pain you feel when you do need to move.

Why does this happen? Besides the stiffening up and pain avoidance response, when muscles are not used, they start to weaken. When you don't continue to put weight on your bones, they lose density and weaken. The nervous system, which interacts with every part of your bodily functions, start to weaken their connection. Are you seeing a pattern here?

Healthy people who begin exercise and/or weight-lifting routines usually go through periods of muscle strain and bone ache as they begin to push their bodies to do more than they previously had. But as they push through and continue, their muscles and organs start to build up to work better together. Even the heart gets healthier as it works to keep up with the extra blood needed to be pumped to feed the level of activity that is now occurring. The capacity of the lungs increases as the demand for oxygen in the blood and to the organs increases to compensate for the healthier, growing masses of muscle and organs working together more efficiently and harmoniously. When you go to move, the body

is better prepared and doesn't give you the pain response in a protective warning.

Wouldn't it be nice to move without the anticipation of your body's bombardment of pain and protest? Of course! Unfortunately, not everyone, especially those suffering from inflammation or other reasons for long periods of inactivity, can just jump right into a strenuous regime of exercise and muscle building. If they were, they probably wouldn't be so desperately trying to find some way to reduce the pain and stress in their lives and bodies. In addition, some forms of strenuous exercise, when not properly done, can actually cause more damage to the body, and potentially increase inflammation with that damage.

Chapter 7: Planning a proper diet plan

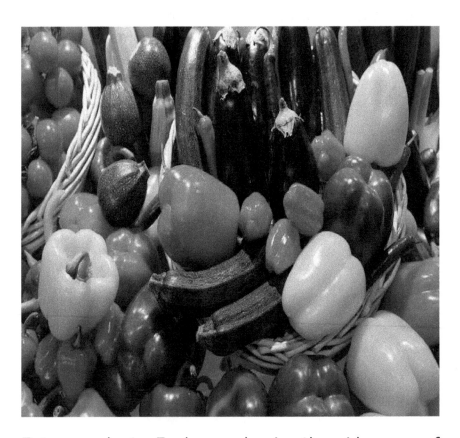

Eat more plants. Explore and enjoy the wide range of fruits and vegetables that provide fiber, antioxidants, and other nutrients to support optimal health. These low-calorie foods combat cellular damage, promote digestion, and help maintain a healthy weight range, which keeps inflammation in check as well.

Discover whole and ancient grains. Ancient grains are those that predate modern varieties created through selective breeding and hybridization—think oats, barley, chia, sorghum, quinoa, bulgur, and the like. These and whole grains retain fiber, antioxidants, and other nutrients that promote a healthy immune response. If whole grains are new to you, try mixing them 50/50 with your usual choice to begin dining the anti-inflammatory way, such as white rice with brown rice, quinoa with couscous, or whole-wheat bread crumbs with white.

Choose healthy fats. Plant-based options like olive oil contain unsaturated fats that support immunity. These are preferable to proinflammatory trans fats and saturated fats from animal products, like butter and bacon. Look for omega-3 fats, such as fish and walnuts, to directly reduce inflammation.

Enjoy nuts and seeds. These little bites provide healthy fats and protein, as well as valuable micronutrients and fiber. Plus, their flavor and crunch enhance any meal or snack.

Add flavor with herbs and spices. Turmeric, ginger, and garlic are anti-inflammatory powerhouses. Have fun exploring these and countless other options for their deep flavors and unique benefits.

Support your microbiome. High-fiber foods like beans and whole grains provide nourishment for your beneficial gut bacteria to thrive. Fermented foods such as yogurt, kimchi, and pickles keep the "communities" of bacteria in your digestive system balanced to help fight inflammation and disease.

Consume power beverages. Coffee and unsweetened black or green tea offer antioxidant compounds that promote resilience against cell damage. Enjoy red wine on occasion, if you like, to maximize anti-inflammatory benefits. Plain water is always a great choice for keeping your body hydrated and energized—vary the flavor and benefits by tossing in some cut fruit or herbs.

Eat fewer processed foods. Highly processed foods are often high in added sugars, refined grains, sodium, and detrimental fats. These types of foods are proinflammatory and also increase one's risk for weight gain and other diseases. If you haven't yet, become a label reader to increase your awareness of what's in these foods—it may surprise and inspire you to run toward the whole foods sections of the store.

Consume less meat. When you want meat, choose and prepare it carefully. Many meats have undesirable amounts of unhealthy fats, and some are pumped full of sodium during processing. Use cooking methods that do not blacken the meat, such as grilling, as the blackened parts that occur have compounds that can contribute to inflammation.

Relax! Stress is a significant contributor to inflammation and disease—in fact, chronic elevation of the stress hormone cortisol leads to ongoing negative impacts on health. Get more sleep, boost your physical activity, and try new activities such as mindfulness meditation—these all help manage stress and keep inflammation down.

Chapter 8: Balancing your Calorie intake

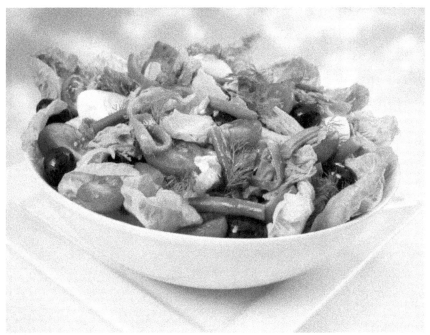

With obesity, for example, a series of causes and effects interact with each other in a downward spiral of declining health. Chronic, low-grade inflammation results directly from consumption of excess calories and obesity. As fat tissue increases, it releases chemicals, hormones, and immune cells that can disrupt normal body function. Proinflammatory cytokines are also released, leading to higher levels of inflammation throughout the body. As the internal system becomes more imbalanced, the risk of developing chronic disorders such as cardiovascular disease, hypertension, type 2 diabetes, and various cancers increases. Many of these conditions increase inflammation themselves. It can become quite complicated when so many of the body's systems are poorly regulated and caught in a feedback loop of actively causing inflammation and damage to other systems.

But there's good news! Consuming anti-inflammatory foods can help straighten out the whole situation, whatever it may be rooted in. An anti-inflammatory diet can support healing if inflammation already exists, and it will provide a foundation for resilience in the future. Shift your focus to this kind of nourishing, balanced, and tasty diet and you'll see a difference in no time, as this diet will restore the energy and sense of well-being you deserve.

Principles of the Anti-Inflammatory Diet

Experts agree that a diet consisting of a wide range of plant-based foods, accompanied by moderate amounts of whole grains, lean proteins, and healthful fats, is the type of eating pattern that will reduce inflammation and ensure a robust immune system. We are constantly learning more about the negative effects of heavily processed, packaged foods, which are often high in inflammation-promoting sodium, added sugars, refined grains, and detrimental fats. Conversely, this book emphasizes fresh, whole foods that are prepared using healthy cooking techniques. Vibrant herbs and spices are not just good for punching up flavor—you'll learn how each brings its own health-supportive qualities to your meals. Prebiotic and probiotic foods support your microbiome—that's the name for the beneficial gut bacteria in your digestive system. These bacteria are linked to a thriving immune system. And you can wash it all down with powerful inflammation-fighting beverages such as unsweetened tea and coffee, water infused with herbs or fruit, and the occasional glass of red wine, if you choose to partake.

We present recipes inspired by the many traditional cuisines around the world that promote a vigorous immune response. Traditional Japanese diets, for instance, are low in fat and full of nutrient-rich vegetables and seafood, but contain very little sugar or refined flour. A modified paleo approach is also explored here, including generous portions of vegetables and hearty protein dishes prepared from the healthiest meats. The Mediterranean eating pattern is well studied for its anti-inflammatory, health-promoting qualities, and many people find its familiar flavors satisfying and appealing. It is based on abundant fruits and vegetables, along with whole grains, legumes, and nuts. Fish, red wine, and olive oil are incorporated regularly in Mediterranean cooking, while red meat, added sugars, and high-fat dairy are limited. We are inspired by this delicious style of eating, so you'll see a lot of recipes here that reflect the Mediterranean approach. But we also recognize that the only anti-inflammatory diet that will work for you is the one you find satisfying and delicious. So after you master the basics, use these principles to figure out which styles you enjoy best and fine-tune your own anti-inflammatory lifestyle path!

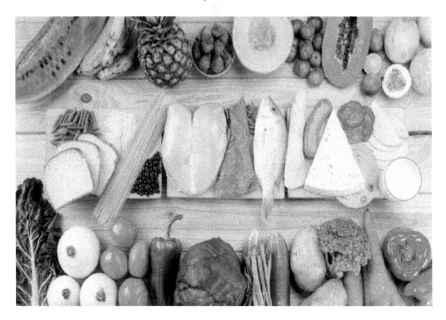

Chapter 9: Breakfast Recipes

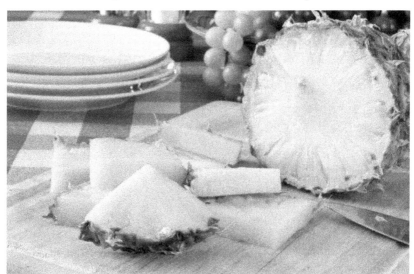

Zucchini and Sprout Breakfast Mix

Preparation time: 10 minutes

Cooking time: 0 minutes

Servings: 4

Ingredients:

2 zucchinis, spiralized

2 cups bean sprouts

4 green onions, chopped

1 red bell pepper, chopped

Juice of 1 lime

1 tablespoon olive oil

½ cup chopped cilantro

¾ cup almonds chopped

A pinch of salt and black pepper

Directions:

In a salad bowl, toss together the zucchinis with the bean sprouts, green onions, bell pepper, cilantro, almonds, salt, pepper, limejuice and oil. Serve for breakfast.

Nutrition Values: calories 140, fat 4, fiber 2, carbs 7, protein 8

Tomato and Olive Salad

Preparation time: 10 minutes

Cooking time: 0 minutes

Servings: 4

Ingredients:

2 cups baby spinach, torn

2 cups cherry tomatoes, halved

4 tablespoons chopped red onion

1 cup chopped cucumber

1 cup kalamata olives, pitted and sliced

1 tablespoon chopped dill

3 tablespoons lemon juice

A pinch of salt and black pepper

2 tablespoons olive oil

Directions:

In a salad bowl, toss the spinach with the tomatoes, onion, cucumber, olives, dill, lemon juice, salt, pepper and oil. Serve for breakfast.

Enjoy!

Nutrition Values: calories 171, fat 2, fiber 5, carbs 11, protein 5

Blueberry and Cashew Mix

Preparation time: 10 minutes

Cooking time: 12 minutes

Servings: 2

Ingredients:

2 bananas, peeled and sliced

¼ cup cashews

¼ cup blueberries

1 tablespoon almond butter

1/3 cup coconut flakes, unsweetened

1 cup coconut milk, unsweetened

Directions:

In a small pot, mix the berries with the coconut flakes, milk, cashews, almond butter and bananas. Mix together and bring to a simmer over medium heat. Cook for 12 minutes, divide into bowls and serve for breakfast.

Enjoy!

Nutrition Values: calories 370, fat 23, fiber 6, carbs 40, protein 8

Easy Almond Zucchini Bowl

Preparation time: 10 minutes

Cooking time: 15 minutes

Servings: 2

Ingredients:

1 cup egg whites, whisked

1½ tablespoons ground flaxseed

1 cup almond milk, unsweetened

1 banana, peeled and mashed

1 small zucchini, grated

½ teaspoon ground cinnamon

Directions:

In a small pan, combine the milk with the egg whites, flaxseed, banana, zucchini and cinnamon powder. Bring to a simmer, mixing constantly, over medium heat. Cook for 15 minutes, divide into bowls and serve for breakfast.

Enjoy!

Nutrition Values: calories 201, fat 6, fiber 9, carbs 14, protein 6

Sweet Potato Hash

Preparation time: 10 minutes

Cooking time: 15 minutes

Servings: 4

Ingredients:

1 sweet potato, peeled and cubed

1 celery root, peeled and cubed

1 cup coconut milk

2 tablespoons olive oil

1 small yellow onion, chopped

1 teaspoon smoked paprika

4 garlic cloves, minced

2 tablespoons parsley, chopped

A pinch of salt and black pepper

Directions:

Heat up a pan with the oil over medium-high heat. Add the celery root and the sweet potato, toss and cook for 5 minutes. Add the onion, garlic, salt, pepper, parsley and paprika then toss and cook for 8 minutes more. Add the coconut milk, mix and cook for 1-2 minutes. Divide everything into bowls and serve for breakfast.

Enjoy!

Nutrition Values: calories 188, fat 2, fiber 8, carbs 10, protein 4

Zucchini Breakfast Salad

Preparation time: 10 minutes

Cooking time: 0 minutes

Servings: 4

Ingredients:

2 zucchinis, spiralized

1 cup beets, baked, peeled and grated

½ bunch kale, chopped

2 tablespoons olive oil

For the tahini sauce:

1 tablespoon maple syrup

Juice of 1 lime

¼ inch fresh ginger, grated

1/3 cup sesame seed paste

Directions:

In a salad bowl, mix the zucchinis with the beets, kale and oil. In another small bowl, whisk the maple syrup with lime juice, ginger and sesame paste. Pour the dressing over the salad, toss and serve it for breakfast.

Enjoy!

Nutrition Values: calories 183, fat 3, fiber 2, carbs 7, protein 9

Quinoa and Spinach Breakfast Salad

Preparation time: 10 minutes

Cooking time: 0 minutes

Servings: 2

Ingredients:

16 ounces quinoa, cooked

1 handful raisins

1 handful baby spinach leaves

1 tablespoon maple syrup

½ tablespoon lemon juice

4 tablespoons olive oil

1 teaspoon ground cumin

A pinch of sea salt and black pepper

½ teaspoon chili flakes

Directions:

In a bowl, mix the quinoa with the spinach, raisins, cumin, salt and pepper and toss. Add the maple syrup, lemon juice, oil and chili flakes and toss then serve for breakfast.

Enjoy!

Nutrition Values: calories 170, fat 3, fiber 6, carbs 8, protein 5

Carrots Breakfast Mix

Preparation time: 10 minutes

Cooking time: 0 minutes

Servings: 4

Ingredients:

1½ tablespoon maple syrup

1 teaspoon olive oil

1 tablespoon chopped walnuts

1 onion, chopped

4 cups shredded carrots

1 tablespoon curry powder

¼ teaspoon ground turmeric

Black pepper to the taste

2 tablespoons sesame seed paste

¼ cup lemon juice

½ cup chopped parsley

Directions:

In a salad bowl, mix together the onion with the carrots, turmeric, curry powder, black pepper, lemon juice and parsley. Add the maple syrup, oil, walnuts and sesame seed paste. toss well and serve for breakfast.

Enjoy!

Nutrition Values: calories 150, fat 3, fiber 2, carbs 6, protein 8

Avocado Omelet

Preparation time: 10 minutes

Cooking time: 10 minutes

Servings: 2

Ingredients:

4 eggs, whisked

2 avocados, pitted, peeled and cubed

A pinch of salt and black pepper

Juice of ½ lemon

1 tablespoon chopped parsley

1 tablespoon olive oil

Directions:

In a bowl, mix the eggs with the avocados, salt, pepper, lemon juice and parsley. Heat up a pan with the oil over medium-high heat then add the avocado and egg mix, spread into the pan and cook for 4 minutes on each side. Divide between plates and serve for breakfast.

Enjoy!

Nutrition Values: calories 201, fat 2, fiber 5, carbs 11, protein 5

Italian Breakfast Salad

Preparation time: 10 minutes

Cooking time: 0 minutes

Servings: 4

Ingredients:

1 handful kalamata olives, pitted and sliced

1 cup cherry tomatoes, halved

1½ cucumbers, sliced

1 red onion, chopped

2 tablespoons chopped oregano

1 tablespoon chopped mint

For the salad dressing:

2 tablespoons balsamic vinegar

¼ cup olive oil

1 garlic clove, minced

2 teaspoons dried Italian herbs

A pinch of salt and black pepper

Directions:

In a salad bowl, toss together the olives with the tomatoes, cucumbers, onion, mint and oregano. In a smaller bowl, whisk the vinegar with the oil, garlic, Italian herbs, salt and pepper. Pour the dressing over the salad, toss and serve for breakfast.

Enjoy!

Nutrition Values: calories 191, fat 10, fiber 3, carbs 13, protein 1

Broccoli and Squash Mix

Preparation time: 10 minutes

Cooking time: 15 minutes

Servings: 4

Ingredients:

4 cups spaghetti squash, peeled, cooked and flesh scrapped out

1½ cups broccoli florets

1 tablespoon olive oil

1 cup coconut milk, unsweetened

1 egg, whisked

1 teaspoon garlic powder

A pinch of salt and black pepper

Directions:

Heat up a pan with the oil over medium-high heat, add the spaghetti squash and the broccoli. Stir and cook for 5-6 minutes. Add the garlic powder, salt, pepper, garlic powder and the egg. Stir and cook for 5 minutes more. Add the coconut milk, mix and cook for about 5 minutes more then divide into bowls and serve for breakfast.

Enjoy!

Nutrition Values: calories 207, fat 5, fiber 8, carbs 14, protein 7

Greens and Berries Mix

Preparation time: 10 minutes

Cooking time: 0 minutes

Servings: 2

Ingredients:

½ cup spinach, torn

½ cup kale, torn

1 cup strawberries, halved

1 cup blueberries

1 banana, peeled and chopped

6 mint leaves, chopped

Directions:

In a bowl, mix the spinach with the kale, strawberries, blueberries, banana and mint. Serve for breakfast.

Enjoy!

Nutrition Values: calories 198, fat 4, fiber 2, carbs 8, protein 6

Veggie and Eggs

Preparation time: 10 minutes

Cooking time: 15 minutes

Servings: 6

Ingredients:

1 red bell pepper, chopped

4 cherry tomatoes, chopped

3 spring onions, chopped

A handful kale, torn

1 tablespoon olive oil

6 eggs

A pinch of salt and black pepper

A pinch of curry powder

Directions:

Heat up a pan with the oil over medium-high heat, add the onions, stir and cook for 1-2 minutes. Add the bell pepper, the tomatoes, the kale, salt, pepper and the curry powder, stir and cook for 4-5 minutes. Crack the eggs into the pan and mix well. Cook until the eggs are done, divide between plates and serve for breakfast.

Enjoy!

Nutrition Values: calories 106, fat 8, fiber 1, carbs 4, protein 7

Coconut Pear Bowl

Preparation time: 10 minutes

Cooking time: 15 minutes

Servings: 4

Ingredients:

2 cups coconut milk, unsweetened

1/3 cup coconut flakes, unsweetened

½ teaspoon vanilla extract

3 pears, peeled, cored and cubed

1. **Directions:**

Put the milk in a small pot, add the coconut, vanilla and pears. Stir and bring to a simmer over medium heat, cook for 15 minutes, divide into bowls and serve.

Enjoy!

Nutrition Values: calories 172, fat 5, fiber 7, carbs 8, protein 4

Breakfast Corn Salad

Preparation time: 10 minutes

Cooking time: 0 minutes

Servings: 4

Ingredients:

2 avocados, pitted, peeled and cubed

1-pint mixed cherry tomatoes, halved

2 cups fresh corn kernels

1 red onion, chopped

For the salad dressing:

2 tablespoons olive oil

1 tablespoon lime juice

½ teaspoon grated lime zest

A pinch of salt and black pepper

¼ cup chopped cilantro

Directions:

In a salad bowl, mix the avocados with the tomatoes, corn and onion. Add the oil, lime juice, lime zest, salt, pepper and the cilantro, toss and serve for breakfast.

Nutrition Values: calories 140, fat 3, fiber 2, carbs 6, protein 9

Simple Basil Tomato Mix

Preparation time: 10 minutes

Cooking time: 0 minutes

Servings: 6

Ingredients:

½ cup extra-virgin olive oil

1 cucumber, chopped

2 pints colored cherry tomatoes, halved

Salt and black pepper to the taste

1 red onion, chopped

3 tablespoons red vinegar

1 garlic clove, minced

1 bunch basil, roughly chopped

Directions:

In a salad bowl, toss together the cucumber with the tomatoes, onion, salt, pepper, oil, vinegar, basil and garlic. Serve for breakfast.

Enjoy!

Nutrition Values: calories 100, fat 1, fiber 2, carbs 2, protein 6

Cucumber and Avocado Salad

Preparation time: 10 minutes

Cooking time: 0 minutes

Servings: 4

Ingredients:

1 pound cucumbers, chopped

2 avocados, pitted and chopped

1 small red onion, thinly sliced

2 tablespoons olive oil

2 tablespoons lemon juice

¼ cup chopped parsley

A pinch of salt and black pepper

Directions:

In a salad bowl, mix together the cucumbers with the avocados, onion, oil, lemon juice, parsley, salt and pepper. Serve for breakfast.

Enjoy!

Nutrition Values: calories 120, fat 2, fiber 2, carbs 3, protein 4

Watermelon Salad

Preparation time: 10 minutes

Cooking time: 0 minutes

Servings: 2

Ingredients:

½ teaspoon agave nectar

2 tablespoons lemon juice

1 tablespoon extra-virgin olive oil

1 jalapeno, seeded and chopped

12 ounces watermelon, chopped

1 red onion, thinly sliced

½ cup chopped basil leaves

2 cups baby arugula

Directions:

In a bowl, toss together the watermelon with the jalapeno, onion, basil, arugula, oil, agave nectar, lemon juice and oil. Serve for breakfast.

Nutrition Values: calories 128, fat 8, fiber 2, carbs 16, protein 2

Coconut Porridge

Preparation time: 10 minutes

Cooking time: 15 minutes

Servings: 2

Ingredients:

2 cups coconut milk, unsweetened

3 tablespoons almond flour

½ cup coconut flakes, unsweetened

2 tablespoons ground flax meal

1 teaspoon vanilla extract

2 teaspoons ground cinnamon

Directions:

In a small pot, mix the coconut milk with the almond flour, coconut flakes, flax meal, vanilla and cinnamon. Stir and bring to a simmer over medium heat for 15 minutes. Divide into bowls and serve for breakfast.

Enjoy!

Nutrition Values: calories 287, fat 5, fiber 7, carbs 13, protein 5

Blackberry and Strawberry Salad

Preparation time: 5 minutes

Cooking time: 0 minutes

Servings: 1

Ingredients:

¼ cup sliced almonds

¼ cup blackberries

¼ cup strawberries, halved

1 banana, peeled and sliced

A pinch of ground cinnamon

Directions:

In a bowl, mix the blackberries with strawberries, cinnamon, banana and almonds. Serve for breakfast.

Enjoy!

Nutrition Values: calories 90, fat 3, fiber 1, carbs 0, protein 5

Breakfast Kale Frittata

Preparation time: 10 minutes

Cooking time: 30 minutes

Servings: 4

Ingredients:

6 kale stalks, chopped

1 small sweet onion, chopped

1 small broccoli head, florets separated

2 garlic cloves, minced

Salt and black pepper to the taste

4 eggs

1 tablespoon olive oil

Directions:

Heat up a pan with the oil over medium-high heat, add the onion, stir and cook for 4-5 minutes. Add the garlic, broccoli and kale, toss and cook for 5 minutes more. Add the eggs, salt and pepper and mix. Place in the oven and bake at 380 degrees F for 20 minutes. Slice and serve for breakfast.

Enjoy!

Nutrition Values: calories 214, fat 7, fiber 2, carbs 12, protein 8

Cranberry Granola Bars

Preparation time: 2 hours

Cooking time: 0 minutes

Servings: 4

Ingredients:

2 cups walnuts, toasted

1 cup dates, pitted

3 tablespoons water

¾ cup cranberries, dried, no added sugar

2 cups desiccated coconut, unsweetened

Directions:

In your food processor, mix dates with coconut, cranberries, water and walnuts. Pulse really well then spread the mix into a lined baking dish. Press well into the dish and keep in the fridge for 2 hours then cut into bars and serve.

Enjoy!

Nutrition Values: calories 476, fat 40, fiber 9, carbs 33, protein 6

Spinach and Berry Smoothie

Preparation time: 10 minutes

Cooking time: 0 minutes

Servings: 2

Ingredients:

1 cup blackberries

1 avocado, pitted, peeled and chopped

1 banana, peeled and roughly chopped

1 cup baby spinach

1 tablespoon hemp seeds

1 cup water

½ cup almond milk, unsweetened

Directions:

In your blender, mix the berries with the avocado, banana, spinach, hemp seeds, water and almond milk. Pulse well, divide into 2 glasses and serve for breakfast.

Enjoy!

Nutrition Values: calories 160, fat 3, fiber 4, carbs 6, protein 3

Chapter 10: Lunch Recipes

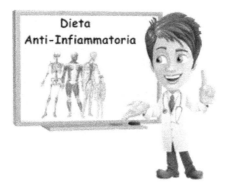

Tasty Grilled Asparagus

Preparation time: 10 minutes

Cooking time: 6 minutes

Servings: 4

Ingredients:

2 pounds asparagus, trimmed

2 tablespoons organic olive oil

A pinch of salt and black pepper

Directions:

In a bowl, combine the asparagus with salt, pepper and oil and toss well.

Place the asparagus on preheated grill over medium-high heat, cook for 3 minutes with them, divide between plates and serve as being a side dish.

Enjoy!

Nutrition Values: calories 172, fat 4, fiber 7, carbs 14, protein 8

Easy Roasted Carrots

Preparation time: ten mins

Cooking time: 30 minutes

Servings: 4

Ingredients:

2 pounds carrots, quartered

A pinch of black pepper

3 tablespoons olive oil

2 tablespoons parsley, chopped

Directions:

Arrange the carrots with a lined baking sheet, add black pepper and oil, toss, introduce inside the oven and cook at 400 degrees F to get a half-hour.

Add parsley, toss, divide between plates and serve as a side dish.

Enjoy!

Nutrition Values: calories 177, fat 3, fiber 6, carbs 14, protein 6

Oven Roasted Asparagus

Preparation time: 10 mins

Cooking time: 25 minutes

Servings: 4

Ingredients:

2 pounds asparagus spears, trimmed

3 tablespoons essential organic olive oil

A pinch of black pepper

2 teaspoons sweet paprika

1 teaspoon sesame seeds

Directions:

Arrange the asparagus on the lined baking sheet, add oil, black pepper and paprika, toss, introduce inside oven and bake at 400 degrees F for 25 minutes.

Divide the asparagus between plates, sprinkle sesame seeds ahead and serve as being a side dish.

Enjoy!

Nutrition Values: calories 190, fat 4, fiber 8, carbs 11, protein 5

Squash Side Salad

Preparation time: 10 minutes

Cooking time: a half-hour

Servings: 6

Ingredients:

1 cup orange juice

3 tablespoons coconut sugar

1 and ½ tablespoons mustard

1 tablespoon ginger, grated

1 and ½ pounds butternut squash, peeled and roughly cubed

Cooking spray

A pinch of black pepper

1/3 cup extra virgin olive oil

6 cups salad greens

1 radicchio, sliced

½ cup pistachios, roasted

Directions:

In a bowl, combine the orange juice with all the sugar, mustard, ginger, black pepper and squash, toss well, spread on a lined baking sheet, spray everything with oil, introduce inside oven and bake at 400 degrees F for thirty minutes.

In a salad bowl, combine the squash with salad greens, radicchio, pistachios and oil, toss well, divide between plates and serve like a side dish.

Enjoy!

Nutrition Values: calories 275, fat 3, fiber 4, carbs 16, protein 6

Colored Iceberg Salad

Preparation time: ten mins

Cooking time: 0 minutes

Servings: 4

Ingredients:

1 iceberg lettuce head, leaves torn

6 bacon slices, cooked and halved

2 green onions, sliced

3 carrots, shredded

6 radishes, sliced

¼ cup red vinegar

¼ cup essential olive oil

3 garlic cloves, minced

A pinch of black pepper

Directions:

In a substantial salad bowl, combine the lettuce leaves with the bacon, green onions, carrots, radishes, vinegar, oil, garlic and black pepper, toss, divide between plates and serve being a side dish.

Enjoy!

Nutrition Values: calories 235, fat 4, fiber 4, carbs 10, protein 6

Fennel Side Salad

Preparation time: ten mins

Cooking time: 0 minutes

Servings: 4

Ingredients:

2 fennel bulbs, trimmed and shaved

1 and ¼ cups zucchini, sliced

2/3 cup dill, chopped

¼ cup freshly squeezed fresh lemon juice

¼ cup essential olive oil

6 cups arugula

½ cups walnuts, chopped

1/3 cup low-fat feta cheese, crumbled

Directions:

In a substantial bowl, combine the fennel while using zucchini, dill, fresh freshly squeezed lemon juice, arugula, oil, walnuts and cheese, toss, divide between plates and serve as a side dish.

Enjoy!

Nutrition Values: calories 188, fat 4, fiber 5, carbs 14, protein 6

Corn Mix

Preparation time: ten minutes

Cooking time: 0 minutes

Servings: 4

Ingredients:

½ cup cider vinegar

¼ cup coconut sugar

A pinch of black pepper

4 cups corn

½ cup red onion, chopped

½ cup cucumber, sliced

½ cup red bell pepper, chopped

½ cup cherry tomatoes, halved

3 tablespoons parsley, chopped

1 tablespoon basil, chopped

1 tablespoon jalapeno, chopped

2 cups baby arugula leaves

Directions:

In a big bowl, combine the corn with onion, cucumber, bell pepper, cherry tomatoes, parsley, basil, jalapeno and arugula and toss.

Add vinegar, sugar and black pepper, toss well, divide between plates and serve just like a side dish.

Enjoy!

Nutrition Values: calories 100, fat 2, fiber 3, carbs 14, protein 4

Persimmon Side Salad

Preparation time: ten mins

Cooking time: 0 minutes

Servings: 4

Ingredients:

Seeds from 1 pomegranate

2 persimmons, cored and sliced

5 cups baby arugula

6 tablespoons green onions, chopped

4 navel oranges, peeled and cut into segments

¼ cup apple cider vinegar

1/3 cup essential olive oil

3 tablespoons pine nuts

1 and ½ teaspoons orange zest, grated

2 tablespoons orange juice

1 tablespoon coconut sugar

½ shallot, chopped

A pinch of cinnamon powder

Directions:

In a salad bowl, combine the pomegranate seeds with persimmons, arugula, green onions and oranges and toss.

In another bowl, combine the vinegar with all the oil, pine nuts, orange zest, orange juice, sugar, shallot and cinnamon, whisk well, add to the salad, toss and serve like a side dish.

Enjoy!

Nutrition Values: calories 188, fat 4, fiber 4, carbs 14, protein 4

Roast green beans with cranberries

Preparation Time: 30 minutes

Servings: 4

Ingredients:

Halved green beans- 2 Ib.

Dried cranberries- ¼ cup

Chopped almonds -¼ cup

Olive oil- 3 tbsp.

Salt

Black pepper

Directions:

Arrange the green beans on a baking sheet and sprinkle oil, salt, and pepper on it.

Mix and roast in the oven for 15 minutes at 425°F.

Stir in the almonds and cranberries and cook for 5 minutes.

Serve.

Nutrition Values:

Calories 181, carbs 10, protein 6, fiber 5, fats 3

Roasted cheesy mushrooms

Preparation Time: 25 minutes

Servings: 4

Ingredients:

Sliced cremini mushrooms- 1½ Ib.

Grated zest of 1 lemon

Grated parmesan - ¼ cup

Dried thyme- 2 tsp.

Minced garlic cloves- 3

Lemon juice- ¼ cup

Olive oil- 3 tbsp.

Salt

Black pepper

Directions:

Coat the baking dish with oil and mix mushrooms with zest, juice, Parmesan, thyme, salt, pepper, and garlic.

Bake in the oven for 15 minutes at 375°F.

Serve.

Nutrition Values:

Calories 199, carbs 12, protein 7, fiber 7, fats 2

Herbed Pork

Preparation time: 10 mins

Cooking time: 60 minutes and 10 minutes

Servings: 6

Ingredients:

2 and ½ pounds pork loin boneless, trimmed and cubed

¾ cup low-sodium chicken stock

2 tablespoons extra virgin extra virgin olive oil

½ tablespoon sweet paprika

2 and ¼ teaspoon sage, dried

½ tablespoon garlic powder

¼ teaspoon rosemary, dried

¼ teaspoon marjoram, dried

1 teaspoon basil, dried

1 teaspoon oregano, dried black pepper

Directions:

In a bowl, mix oil with stock, paprika, garlic powder, sage, rosemary, thyme, marjoram, oregano and pepper for the taste and whisk well.

Heat up a pan over medium-high heat, add the pork and brown it for 5 minutes on either sides.

Add the herbed mix, toss well, cook over medium heat for an hour, divide between plates and serve employing a side salad.

Enjoy!

Nutrition Values: calories 310, fat 4, fiber 6, carbs 12, protein 14

Garlic Pork Shoulder

Preparation time: 10 mins

Cooking time: 4 hours and thirty minutes

Servings: 6

Ingredients:

3 tablespoons garlic, minced

3 tablespoons extra virgin essential olive oil

4 pounds pork shoulder

2 teaspoons sweet paprika

Black pepper for the taste

Directions:

In a bowl, mix extra virgin extra virgin olive oil with paprika, black pepper and oil and whisk well.

Brush pork shoulder with this mix, arrange inside a baking dish and introduce inside oven at 425 degrees for twenty or so minutes.

Reduce heat to 325 degrees F and bake for 4 hours.

Slice the meat, divide it between plates and serve having a side salad.

Enjoy!

Nutrition Values: calories 321, fat 6, fiber 4, carbs 12, protein 18

Pork and Creamy Veggie Sauce

Preparation time: 10 mins

Cooking time: one hour and twenty approximately minutes

Servings: 4

Ingredients:

2 pounds pork roast

1 cup low-sodium veggie stock

2 carrots, chopped

1 leek, chopped

1 celery stalk, chopped

1 teaspoon black peppercorns

2 yellow onions, cut into quarters

1 tablespoon chives, chopped

1 tablespoon parsley, chopped

2 cups nonfat yogurt

1 cup coconut cream

1 teaspoon mustard

Black pepper towards the taste

Directions:

Put the roast in a baking dish, add carrots, leek, celery, peppercorns, onions, stock and black pepper, cover, introduce inside oven and bake at 400 degrees F for sixty minutes and 10 minutes

Transfer the roast using a platter and all sorts of the veggies mix with a pan.

Heat this mix over medium heat, add yogurt, cream and mustard, toss, cook for ten mins, drizzle inside the roast and serve.

Enjoy!

Nutrition Values: calories 263, fat 4, fiber 2, carbs 12, protein 22

Ground Pork Pan

Preparation Time: 10 mins

Cooking time: 20 mins

Servings: 4

Ingredients:

Zest of merely one lemon, grated

Juice of a single lemon

2 garlic cloves, minced

1 tablespoon organic olive oil

1 pound pork meat, ground

Black pepper on the taste

1-pint cherry tomatoes, chopped

1 small red onion, chopped

½ cup low-sodium veggie stock,

2 tablespoons low-sodium tomato paste

1 tablespoon basil, chopped

Directions:

Heat up a pan with all the oil over medium heat, add garlic and onion, stir and cook for 5 minutes.

Add pork, black pepper, tomatoes, stock, freshly squeezed freshly squeezed lemon juice, lemon zest and tomato paste, toss and cook for quarter-hour.

Add basil, toss, divide between plates and serve.

Enjoy!

Nutrition Values: calories 286, fat 8, fiber 7, carbs 14, protein 17

Tarragon Pork Steak

Preparation time: 10 minutes

Cooking time: 22 minutes

Servings: 4

Ingredients:

4 medium pork steaks

Black pepper towards the taste

1 tablespoon extra virgin olive oil

8 cherry tomatoes, halved

A handful tarragon, chopped

Directions:

Heat up a pan while using the oil over medium-high heat, add steaks, season with black pepper, cook them for 6 minutes on each side and divide between plates.

Heat the same pan over medium heat, add the tomatoes along with the tarragon, cook for ten minutes, divide next around the pork and serve.

Enjoy!

Nutrition Values: calories 263, fat 4, fiber 6, carbs 12, protein 16

Pork Meatballs

Preparation time: ten minutes

Cooking time: 10 mins

Servings: 4

Ingredients:

1 pound pork, ground

1/3 cup cilantro, chopped

1 cup red onion, chopped

4 garlic cloves, minced

1 tablespoon ginger, grated

1 Thai chili, chopped

2 tablespoons extra virgin olive oil

Directions:

In a bowl, combine the meat with cilantro, onion, garlic, ginger and chili, stir well and shape medium meatballs out of this mix.

Heat up a pan while using oil over medium-high heat, add the meatballs, cook them for 5 minutes on either side, divide them between plates and serve with a side salad.

Enjoy!

Nutrition Values: calories 220, fat 4, fiber 2, carbs 8, protein 14

Nutmeg Meatballs Curry

Preparation Time: 40 minutes

Servings: 3

Ingredients:

Pork meat, ground- 2/3 lbs.

Egg -½

Parsley, chopped-1 tbsp

Coconut flour-2 tbsp

Garlic clove, minced-1

Salt and black pepper - to taste

Veggie stock -¼ cup

Tomato passata-½ cup

Nutmeg, ground -¼ tsp

Sweet paprika -¼ tsp

Olive oil-1 tbsp

Carrot, chopped -1

Directions:

Thoroughly mix the meat with egg, parsley, salt, pepper, garlic, nutmeg, and paprika in a suitable bowl.

Mix well and make small meatballs out of this mixture.

Dredge these balls through dry flour or dust the balls with flour.

Place a pot with oil over medium-high heat.

Add dusted meatballs in the pot and sear them for 4 minutes per side.

Toss in tomato passata, carrots, and stock.

Cover this mixture and let it simmer for 20 minutes.

Serve right away.

Devour.

Nutrition Values:

Calories: 281, Fat: 8, Fiber: 6, Carbs: 10, Protein: 15

Pan seared sausage and kale

Preparation Time: 35 minutes

Servings: 4

Ingredients:

Chopped kale- 5 Ib.

Italian pork sausage: sliced- 1½ Ib.

Minced garlic- 1 tsp.

Water- 1 cup

Onion: chopped- 1 cup

Red bell pepper: seeded and chopped ½ cup

Red chili pepper: chopped ½ cup

Black pepper

Salt

Directions:

Put a pan on medium heat and add the sausage to brown for 10 minutes.

Mix in onions and town for 3-4 minutes.

Add in the garlic and bell pepper and cook for 1 minute.

Mix in the chili, kale, water, pepper and salt and let cook for 10 minutes.

Serve

Nutrition Values:

Calories- 872, carbs- 61, protein- 54, fiber- 3, fats- 43

Pan-Fried Chorizo Mix

Preparation Time: 35 minutes

Servings: 4

Ingredients:

Chopped tomato, 1

Olive oil, 1 tbsp.

Sugar-free chorizo sausages, 2

Chopped zucchini, 1

Chopped red bell pepper, 1

Minced garlic cloves, 2

Black pepper

Chicken stock, 2 cup.

Chopped parsley, 2 tbsps.

Lemon juice, 1 tbsp.

Salt

Chopped yellow onion, 1

Directions:

Set the pan on fire to fry the chorizo and onion for 3 minutes over medium-high heat.

Stir in the bell pepper, garlic, lemon juice, tomato, pepper, stock, and salt.

Allow to simmer for 10 minutes while covered

Mix in the zucchini and parsley to cook for 12 minutes.

Set in serving bowls and enjoy

Nutrition Values:

Calories: 280, Fat: 8, Fiber: 3, Carbs: 5, Protein: 17

Pork Rolls

Preparation Time: 30 minutes

Servings: 6

Ingredients:

3 Peeled and minced garlic cloves

Italian seasoning - ½ teaspoon

6 prosciutto slices

Chopped fresh parsley - 2 tablespoons

Thinly sliced pork cutlets- 1 pound

Coconut oil - 1 tablespoon

Chopped onion- ¼ cup

Canned diced tomatoes - 15 ounces

Chicken stock - ⅓ cup

Grated Parmesan cheese - 2 tablespoons

Ricotta cheese- ⅓ cup e

Seasoning: Salt and ground black pepper

Directions:

Flatten pork pieces with a meat pounder.

Put prosciutto slices on top of each piece and then divide ricotta cheese, parsley, and Parmesan cheese.

Each piece of pork should be rolled and secure with a toothpick.

With medium-high temperature, heat the oil in a pan, add pork rolls, cook until brown on both sides, and transfer to a plate.

Heat the pan again over medium temperature, put onion and garlic, mix well. Cook for 5 minutes.

The stock should be added and cook for another 3 minutes.

Remove toothpicks from pork rolls and return into the pan.

Put tomatoes, Italian seasoning, salt, and pepper, bring to commotion by stirring, bring to a boil, reduce heat to medium-low, cover the pan with lid, and cook for 30 minutes.

Divide between plates and serve it.

Nutrition Values:

Calories: 256, Fat: 19, Fiber: 1, Carbs: 17, Protein: 12

Salad Bowl of CapreseWith Tomato

Preparation Time: 7 minutes

Servings: 3

Ingredients:

Mozzarella cheese-1/2 pound (sliced)

Balsamic vinegar-1 tablespoon

Olive oil-1 tablespoon

Tomato-1 (sliced)

Basil leaves-4 (torn)

Salt and black pepper-To taste

Instructions:

Settle the tomato and mozzarella slices alternatively.

Display on 2 plates. Season with the salt and pepper.

Drizzle the vinegar and olive oil. Sprinkle the basil leaves at the end.

Serve.

Nutrition :

Calories:- 150; Fat : 12; Fiber : 5; Carbs : 6; Protein : 9

Sauté Cabbage with Butter

Preparation and Cooking Time 20 minutes.

Servings: 4

Ingredients:

Green cabbage, shredded: 1½ pound

Salt: to taste

Ground black pepper: to taste

Unsalted butter: 5 ounces

Sweet paprika: 1/8 teaspoon

Directions:

Place a medium skillet pan over medium heat, add butter and when it melts, add cabbage.

Cook cabbage for 15 minutes, stirring often and then season with salt, black pepper, and paprika.

Continue cooking for 1 minute, then divide evenly between plates and serve.

Nutrition Values:

Calories: 805, Fat: 84, Fiber: 3, Carbs: 9, Protein: 1

Saute Edamame with Mint

Preparation and Cooking Time 10 minutes

Servings: 4

Ingredients:

Edamame: ¾ pound

Salt: to taste

Ground black pepper: to taste

Mint leaves, chopped: 1 tablespoon

Olive oil: 2 teaspoons

Green onions, chopped: 3

Minced garlic: ½ teaspoon

Directions:

Place a pan over medium heat, add oil and when hot, add edamame beans.

Season with salt and black pepper, then add remaining ingredients and stir until well mixed.

Cook edamame for 5 minutes until heated through, then divide evenly between serving plates and serve.

Nutrition Values:

Calories: 91, Fat: 3, Fiber: 4, Carbs: 17, Protein: 7

Sauteed Broccoli with Parmesan

Preparation Time: 32 minutes

Servings: 4

Ingredients:

broccoli florets - 1 pound

garlic clove - 1, minced

parmesan - 1 tablespoon, grated

olive oil - 5 tablespoons

Salt and black pepper to the taste.

Instructions:

Pour some water in a pot, then add a little salt and bring to a boil over medium high heat source.

Then add broccoli, cook for 5 minutes before removing the water.

Heat up a pan containing the oil over medium high heat source; then add garlic. Stir and cook for about 2 more minutes

Add broccoli; stir and cook for another 15 minutes

Remove the heat; sprinkle parmesan.

Divide into clean plates and serve

Nutrition :

Calories:- 193; Fat : 14; Fiber : 3; Carbs : 6; Protein : 5

Sautéed Kohlrabi with Parsley

Preparation and Cooking Time 15 minutes

Servings: 4

Ingredients:

Kohlrabi, trimmed and sliced thin: 2

Salt: to taste

Ground black pepper: to taste

Chopped parsley: 1 tablespoon

Unsalted butter: 1 tablespoon

Minced garlic: 1 teaspoon

Directions:

Place kohlrabi in a medium saucepan, pour in enough water to cover it, then place the pan over medium heat and bring to boil.

Then cook for 5 minutes, drain kohlrabi and transfer into a bowl.

Place a medium skillet pan over medium heat, add butter and when it melts, add garlic and cook for 1 minute or until fragrant.

Add kohlrabi, season with salt and black pepper and cook for 3 minutes per side or until nicely golden brown on both sides.

Add parsley, toss until mixed and remove pan from heat.

Divide kohlrabi evenly between serving plates and serve straight away.

Nutrition Values:

Calories: 55, Fat: 3, Fiber: 7, Carbs: 8, Protein: 9

Sautéed Mixed Vegetable with Pumpkin Seeds

Preparation and Cooking Time 10 minutes

Servings: 4

Ingredients:

Mushrooms, sliced: 14 ounces

Broccoli florets: 3 ounces

Red bell pepper, seeded and cut into strips: 3 ounces

Spinach, torn: 3 ounces

Garlic, minced: 2 tablespoons

Salt: to taste

Ground black pepper: to taste

Red pepper flakes: 1/8 teaspoon

Olive oil: 6 tablespoons

Pumpkin seeds: 2 tablespoons

Directions:

Place a skillet pan over medium-high heat, add oil and when hot, add garlic and cook for 1 minute or until fragrant.

Add mushrooms and cook for 3 minutes.

Then add broccoli florets and pepper, stir well, season with salt and black pepper, add pepper flakes and pumpkin seeds and cook for 3 minutes.

Add spinach, stir until just mixed, cook for 3 minutes and remove the pan from heat.

Serve straightaway.

Nutrition Values:

Calories: 271, Fat: 27, Fiber: 5, Carbs: 14, Protein: 6

Side Cauliflower Salad

Preparation Time: 15 minutes

Servings: 10

Ingredients:

Mayonnaise. 1 c

Salt

Chopped hard-boiled eggs, 4

Black pepper

Chopped celery, 1 cup.

Cauliflower florets, 21 oz.

Cider vinegar, 2 tbsps.

Erythritol, 1 tsp.

Water, 1 tbsp.

Chopped onion, 1 cup.

Directions:

Microwave the cauliflower florets with water in a heatproof bowl for 5 minutes

Set the salad in a bowl

Mix in the onions, celery, and eggs as you stir gently.

Combine salt, mayonnaise, pepper, vinegar, and erythritol in another bowl.

Add the mixture to the cauliflower, toss and enjoy.

Nutrition Values:

Calories: 139, Fat: 7, Fiber: 9, Carbs: 18, Protein: 8

Spicy Green Beans and Vinaigrette

Preparation Time: 22 minutes

Servings: 8

Ingredients:

Minced garlic clove, 1

Macadamia nut oil, 4 tbsps.

Lemon juice, 1 tsp.

Green beans, 2 lbs.

Smoked paprika, 2 tsps.

Salt

Chopped chorizo, 2 oz.

Black pepper

Coconut oil, 2 tbsps.

Coriander, ¼ tsp.

Beef stock, 2 tbsps.

Coconut vinegar, ½ cup.

Directions:

Put lemon juice, chorizo, vinegar, pepper, paprika, garlic, and salt in a blender to pulse until smooth.

Mix in macadamia nut oil and stock to blend again

Allow the coconut oil to melt over medium heat to sauté the green beans and chorizo mixture.

Cook for 10 minutes as you stir gently

Enjoy this wonderful meal

Nutrition Values:

Calories: 159, Fat: 11, Fiber: 1, Carbs: 8, Protein: 9

Stuffed Sausage with Bacon Wrappings

Preparation Time: 40 minutes

Servings: 4

Ingredients:

Onion powder

Bacon strips,

Salt.

Garlic powder.

Black pepper.

Sausages,

Sweet paprika, ½ tsp.

Pepper jack cheese slices, 1

Directions:

Ensure you have a medium high source of heat. Set a grill on it. Add sausages to cook until done all sides and set on a plate to cool.

Slice a pocket opening in the sausages. Each to be stuffed with 2 slices of pepper jack cheese. Apply a seasoning of onion, pepper, garlic powder, paprika and salt.

Each stuffed sausage should be wrapped in a bacon strip and grip using a toothpick. Set them on the baking sheet and transfer to the oven to bake at 400 0F for almost 15 minutes.

Serve immediately and enjoy.

Nutrition :

calories: 500, fat: 37, fiber: 12, carbs: 4, protein: 40

Tasty Lunch Pizza

Preparation Time: 17 minutes

Servings: 4

Ingredients:

Mascarpone cheese, ¼ cup.

Clive oil, 1 tbsp.

Shredded pizza cheese mix, 1 cup.

Ghee, 2 tbsps.

Heavy cream, 1 tbsp.

Lemon pepper

Shredded mozzarella cheese, 1 cup.

Steamed broccoli florets, 1/3 cup.

Salt.

Minced garlic, 1 tsp.

Black pepper.

Shaved asiago cheese

Directions:

Set the pan on fire to heat the oil to cook pizza mix then spread into a circle over medium heat

Spread the mozzarella cheese into a circle also

Allow everything to cook for 5 minutes and set on a plate

Set the pan on fire to melt the ghee for cooking lemon pepper, mascarpone cheese, cream, salt, pepper, and garlic for 5 minutes over medium heat.

Spread half of this mix over cheese crust.

Mix in broccoli florets to the pan with the remaining mascarpone mix to cook for 1 minute

Top the mixture on the pizza, sprinkle asiago cheese at the end and serve

Nutritional :

calories: 250, fat: 15, fiber: 1, carbs: 3, protein: 10

Turkey and Collard Greens Soup

Preparation and Cooking Time 2 hours and 30 minutes

Servings: 10

Ingredients:

Collard greens, chopped: 5 bunches

Salt: to taste

Ground black pepper: to taste

Red pepper flakes: 1 tablespoon

Chicken stock: 5 cups

Turkey leg: 1

Minced garlic: 2 tablespoons

Olive oil: ¼ cup

Directions:

Place a large pot over medium heat, add oil and when hot, add garlic.

Cook garlic for 1 minute, then turkey, season with salt and black pepper and then pout in stock.

Stir the mixture and simmer the soup for 30 minutes, covering the pot.

Add collard greens, stir until just mixed and cook for 45 minutes, covering the pot.

Then reduce heat to medium level, taste soup to adjust seasoning and continue cooking for 1 hour, covering the pot.

When done, take out greens from the soup using a slotted spoon, then take out the chicken and transfer to a cutting board.

Let the turkey cool for 10 minutes, then chop into bite size pieces and add into the soup.

Return greens into the soup, season with red pepper flakes and ladle evenly into serving bowls.

Serve immediately.

Nutrition Values:

Calories: 171, Fat: 19, Fiber: 8, Carbs: 2, Protein: 11

Warm Delicious Roasted Olives

Preparation Time: 30 minutes

Servings: 6

Ingredients:

kalamata olives - 1 cup, pitted

black olives - 1 cup, pitted

garlic cloves - 10

herbs de Provence - 1 tablespoon

lemon zest - 1 teaspoon, grated

green olives - 1 cup, stuffed with almonds and garlic

olive oil - 1/4 cup

Black pepper to the taste.

Some chopped thyme for serving

Instructions:

Spread black, kalamata and green olives on a lined baking sheet neatly, and drizzle some oil on them as well as on garlic and herbs de Provence,

Then toss to keep it well coated. Transfer into an oven set at a temperature of 425 0F and bake for 10 minutes

Stir the olives and bake for 10 another minutes.

Cut the olives on different plates, sprinkle lemon zest, black pepper and thyme on top.

Toss to ensure it is coated. Serve warm.

Nutrition :

Calories:- 200; Fat : 20; Fiber : 4; Carbs : 3; Protein : 1

Yummy Creamy Spaghetti Pasta: Side Dish

Preparation Time: 50 minutes

Servings: 4

Ingredients:

spaghetti squash - 1

ghee - 2 tablespoons

heavy cream - 2 cups

Cajun seasoning - 1 teaspoon

A pinch of cayenne pepper

Salt and black pepper to the taste.

Instructions:

Prick spaghetti with a fork, then arrange neatly on a lined baking sheet.

Move to an oven at 350 0F and bake for 15 minutes

Remove the spaghetti squash from the oven, keep it aside for a while and let it cool down. Scoop squash noodles

Heat up a pan contalning ghee over medium heat; before adding spaghetti squash.

Then stir gently and cook for a couple of minutes

Sprinkle a pinch of salt, pepper, cayenne pepper and Cajun seasoning.

Then stir and cook for about a minute

Add heavy cream; stir, cook for 10 another 10 minutes.

Cut into different plates and serve as a keto side dish.

Nutrition :

Calories:- 200; Fat : 2; Fiber : 1; Carbs : 5; Protein : 8

Yummy Muffins

Preparation Time: 55 minutes

Servings: 13

Ingredients:

Egg yolks, 6

Coconut flour, ¾ cup.

Mushrooms, ½ lb.

Salt.

Ground beef, 1 lb.

Coconut aminos, 2 tbsps.

Directions:

Combine egg yolks, coconut aminos and salt in a blender. Process well until the desired consistency is attained.

In a separate bowl, stir in salt and beef. Stir in mushroom mixture to combine.

Stir in coconut flour.

Set the mixture into 13 cupcake cups and transfer into an oven preheated at 350 0F. bake the cups until done for 45 minutes

Allow to cool and enjoy your lunch

Nutritional :

calories: 160, fiber: 3, carbs: 1, fat: 10, protein: 12

Zucchini and Squash Noodles with Peppers

Preparation and Cooking Time 30 minutes

Servings: 6

Ingredients:

Medium zucchinis, cut with a spiralizer: 1 ½

Medium summer squash, cut with a spiralizer: 1

Butternut squash, cut with a spiralizer: 4 ounce

Medium white onion, peeled and chopped: 4 ounces

Mixed bell peppers, seeded and cut into thin strips: 6 ounces

Minced garlic: 1 ½ teaspoon

Salt: to taste

Ground black pepper: to taste

Bacon fat: 4 tablespoons

Directions:

Set oven to 400 0F and let preheat.

In the meantime, place zucchini noodles on a baking sheet lined with parchment paper and then add onion and bell peppers.

Add garlic, season with salt and black pepper and toss until evenly coated.

Add bacon fat, toss until coated and place the baking sheet into an oven.

Bake for 20 minutes or until done and serve straightaway.

Nutrition Values:

Calories: 179, Fat: 6, Fiber: 6, Carbs: 19, Protein: 10

Baked Potato Mix

Preparation time: 10 mins

Cooking time: one hour and quarter-hour

Servings: 8

Ingredients:

6 potatoes, peeled and sliced

2 garlic cloves, minced

2 tablespoons organic olive oil

1 and ½ cups coconut cream

¼ cup coconut milk

1 tablespoon thyme, chopped

¼ teaspoon nutmeg, ground

A pinch of red pepper flakes

1 and ½ cups low-fat cheddar, shredded

½ cup low-fat parmesan, grated

Directions:

Heat up a pan with all the oil over medium heat, add garlic, stir and cook for 1 minute.

Add coconut cream, coconut milk, thyme, nutmeg and pepper flakes, stir, bring which has a simmer, reduce heat to low and cook for 10 mins.

Arrange 1/3 with all the potatoes in a very baking dish, add 1/3 with the cream, repeat with the rest through the potatoes along with the cream, sprinkle the cheddar for the top, cover with tin foil, introduce within the oven and cook at 375 degrees F for 45 minutes.

Uncover the dish, sprinkle the parmesan, bake everything for 20 mins, divide between plates and serve as as being a side dish.

Enjoy!

Nutrition Values: calories 224, fat 8, fiber 9, carbs 16, protein 15

Spicy Brussels sprouts

Preparation time: ten mins

Cooking time: 20 minutes

Servings: 6

Ingredients:

2 pounds Brussels sprouts, halved

2 tablespoons essential extra virgin olive oil

A pinch of black pepper

1 tablespoon sesame oil

2 garlic cloves, minced

½ cup coconut aminos

2 teaspoons apple cider vinegar treatment

1 tablespoon coconut sugar

2 teaspoons chili sauce

A pinch of red pepper flakes

Sesame seeds for serving

Directions:

Spread the sprouts over the lined baking dish, add the primary essential olive oil, the sesame oil, black pepper, garlic, aminos, vinegar, coconut sugar, chili sauce and pepper flakes, toss well, introduce within the oven and bake at 425 degrees F for twenty minutes.

Divide the sprouts between plates, sprinkle sesame seeds at the very top and serve as a side dish.

Enjoy!

Nutrition Values: calories 176, fat 3, fiber 6, carbs 14, protein 9

Baked Cauliflower

Preparation time: ten minutes

Cooking time: half an hour

Servings: 4

Ingredients:

3 tablespoons organic extra virgin olive oil

2 tablespoons chili sauce

Juice of a single lime

3 garlic cloves, minced

1 cauliflower head, florets separated

A pinch of black pepper

1 teaspoon cilantro, chopped

Directions:

In a bowl, combine the oil while using chili sauce, lime juice, garlic and black pepper and whisk.

Add cauliflower florets, toss, spread on the lined baking sheet, introduce inside oven and bake at 425 degrees F for a half-hour.

Divide the cauliflower between plates, sprinkle cilantro at the top and serve as being a side dish.

Enjoy!

Nutrition Values: calories 188, fat 4, fiber 7, carbs 14, protein 8

Baked Broccoli

Preparation time: ten minutes

Cooking time: quarter-hour

Servings: 4

Ingredients:

1 tablespoon organic olive oil

1 broccoli head, florets separated

2 garlic cloves, minced

½ cup coconut cream

½ cup low-fat mozzarella, shredded

¼ cup low-fat parmesan, grated

A pinch of pepper flakes, crushed

Directions:

In a baking dish, combine the broccoli with oil, garlic, cream, pepper flakes and mozzarella and toss.

Sprinkle the parmesan on top, introduce inside the oven and bake at 375 degrees F for fifteen minutes.

Divide between plates and serve as a side dish.

Enjoy!

Nutrition Values: calories 188, fat 4, fiber 7, carbs 14, protein 7

Easy Slow Cooked Potatoes

Preparation time: 10 mins

Cooking time: 6 hours

Servings: 6

Ingredients:

Cooking spray

2 pounds baby potatoes, quartered

3 cups low-fat cheddar cheese, shredded

2 garlic cloves, minced

8 bacon slices, cooked and chopped

¼ cup green onions, chopped

1 tablespoon sweet paprika

A pinch of black pepper

Directions:

Spray a pokey cooker while using cooking spray, add baby potatoes, cheddar, garlic, bacon, green onions, paprika and black pepper, toss, cover and cook on High for 6 hours.

Divide between plates and serve being a side dish.

Enjoy!

Nutrition Values: calories 200, fat 4, fiber 6, carbs 12, protein 7

Mashed Potatoes

Preparation time: 10 minutes

Cooking time: 20 mins

Servings: 6

Ingredients:

3 pounds potatoes, peeled and cubed

2 tablespoons non-fat butter

½ cup coconut milk

A pinch of salt and black pepper

½ cup low-fat sour cream

Directions:

Put the potatoes in the pot, add water to purchase, put in a pinch of salt and pepper, bring with a boil over medium heat, cook for twenty or so minutes and drain.

Add butter, milk and sour cream, mash well, stir everything, divide between plates and serve as a side dish.

Enjoy!

Nutrition Values: calories 188, fat 3, fiber 7, carbs 14, protein 8

Avocado Side Salad

Preparation time: ten mins

Cooking time: 0 minutes

Servings: 4

Ingredients:

4 blood oranges, peeled and cut into segments

2 tablespoons extra virgin olive oil

A pinch of red pepper, crushed

2 avocados, peeled, pitted and cut into wedges

1 and ½ cups baby arugula

¼ cup almonds, toasted and chopped

1 tablespoon fresh freshly squeezed lemon juice

Directions:

In a bowl, combine the oranges while using oil, red pepper, avocados, arugula, almonds and fresh lemon juice, toss, divide between plates and serve as being a side dish.

Enjoy!

Nutrition Values: calories 231, fat 4, fiber 8, carbs 16, protein 6

Classic Side Dish Salad

Preparation time: ten mins

Cooking time: 0 minutes

Servings: 4

Ingredients:

3 garlic cloves, minced

Juice of ½ lemon

6 ounces coconut cream

2 lettuce hearts, torn

1 cup corn

4 ounces green beans, halved

1 cup cherry tomatoes, halved

1 cucumber, chopped

1/3 cup chives, chopped

1 avocado, peeled, pitted and halved

6 bacon slices, cooked and chopped

Directions:

In a bowl, combine the lettuce with corn, green beans, cherry tomatoes, cucumber, chives, avocado and bacon and toss.

In another bowl, combine the garlic with fresh fresh lemon juice and coconut cream, whisk well, add towards the salad, toss and serve as a side dish.

Enjoy!

Nutrition Values: calories 175, fat 12, fiber 4, carbs 13, protein 6

Easy Kale Mix

Preparation time: ten mins

Cooking time: 0 minutes

Servings: 4

Ingredients:

1 wheat grains bread slice, toasted and torn into small pieces

6 tablespoons low-fat cheddar, grated

3 tablespoons extra virgin olive oil

5 tablespoons fresh lemon juice

1 garlic herb, minced

7 cups kale, torn

A pinch of black pepper

Directions:

In a bowl, combine the bread with cheese and kale.

In another bowl, combine the oil with all the freshly squeezed lemon juice, garlic and black pepper, whisk, add towards the salad, toss, divide between plates and serve as as a side dish.

Enjoy!

Nutrition Values: calories 200, fat 4, fiber 5, carbs 14, protein 8

Asparagus Salad

Preparation time: ten mins

Cooking time: 4 minutes

Servings: 4

Ingredients:

4 tablespoons avocado oil

2 tablespoons balsamic vinegar

1 tablespoon coconut aminos

1 garlic herb, minced

1 pound asparagus, trimmed

6 cups frisee lettuce leaves, torn

1 cup edamame, shelled

1 cup parsley, chopped

Directions:

Heat up a pan with 1 tablespoon oil over medium-high heat, add asparagus, cook for 4 minutes and transfer which has a salad bowl.

Add lettuce, edammae and parsley and toss.

In another bowl, combine the remaining from your oil when using vinegar, aminos and garlic, whisk well, add inside the salad, toss, divide between plates and serve as being a side dish.

Enjoy!

Nutrition Values: calories 200, fat 4, fiber 5, carbs 14, protein 6

Green Side Salad

Preparation time: 10 minutes

Cooking time: 0 minutes

Servings: 4

Ingredients:

4 cups baby spinach leaves

1 cucumber, sliced

3 ounces broccoli florets

3 ounces green beans, blanched and halved

¾ cup edamame, shelled

1 and ½ cups green grapes, halved

1 cup orange juice

¼ cup extra virgin organic olive oil

1 tablespoon cider vinegar

2 tablespoons parsley, chopped

2 teaspoons mustard

A pinch of black pepper

Directions:

In a salad bowl, combine a baby spinach with cucumber, broccoli, green beans, edamame and grapes and toss.

Add orange juice, organic extra virgin olive oil, vinegar, parsley, mustard and black pepper, toss well, divide between plates and serve as a side dish.

Enjoy!

Nutrition Values: calories 117, fat 4, fiber 5, carbs 14, protein 4

Baked Zucchini

Preparation time: ten mins

Cooking time: 20 minutes

Servings: 4

Ingredients:

4 zucchinis, quartered lengthwise

½ teaspoon thyme, dried

½ teaspoon oregano, dried

½ cup low-fat parmesan, grated

½ teaspoon basil, dried

¼ teaspoon garlic powder

2 tablespoons essential olive oil

2 tablespoons parsley, chopped

A pinch of black pepper

Directions:

Arrange zucchini pieces having a lined baking sheet, add thyme, oregano, basil, garlic powder, oil, parsley and black pepper and toss well.

Sprinkle parmesan ahead, introduce within the oven and bake at 350 degrees F for twenty roughly minutes.

Divide between plates and serve as a side dish.

Enjoy!

Nutrition Values: calories 198, fat 4, fiber 4, carbs 14, protein 5

CONCLUSION

Although the anti-inflammatory diet is generally good for health, it is especially suitable for treating some health problems. For example, the anti-inflammatory diet reduces the risk of heart disease, keeps existing heart problems under control, reduces blood pressure and triglycerides in the blood (natural fats formed by the combination of fatty acids and glycerol) and soothes hard rheumatic joints.

This diet aims to increase physical and mental health by recommending healthy, fat, fiber-rich fruits and vegetables, abundant water, and a limited amount of animal protein (excluding fish), providing a constant source of energy and reducing the risk of age-related diseases.

Good luck!

2

The Affordable Air Fryer Cookbook

The Ultimate Cookbook with 200 Delicious and Easy Recipes For People On a Budget

By Melissa William

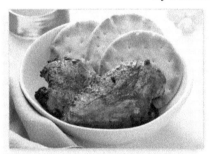 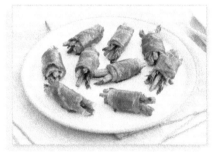

circumstances will any legal responsibility or blame be held against the publisher for any reparation, damages, or monetary loss due to the information herein, either directly or indirectly. Respective authors own all copyrights not held by the publisher.

The information herein is offered for informational purposes solely and is universal as so. The presentation of the information is without contract or any type of guarantee assurance.

The trademarks that are used are without any consent and the publication of the trademark is without permission or backing by the trademark owner. All trademarks and brands within this book are for clarifying purposes only and are the owned by the owners themselves s, not affiliated with this document.

Introduction

Your tongue may have an affection for crispy fried food. But the arteries of yours? Not really. Excessive consumption of fried foods may lead to many diseases.

An air fryer is not just a regular fryer. It's like an oven fryer; it doesn't cook food as pan-frying or deep-frying would. It's essentially a small convection oven with a hot air chamber. It cooks the food a little quicker, spreads heat more equally in the perforated basket in which food is placed. Air fryer speeds up the cooking process, when one is in a hurry and needs to cook a delicious, healthy meal, to save you from all the trouble of waiting, there is an air fryer. The term fry always comes up with deep frying because they get food crispy while frying them and the opposite mechanism is with air fryers because they're not traditional fryers, and oil is not used to get the food crisp and healthy.

It is one of the healthiest methods to cook crispy and fried food. You can cook anything from baked seeds to moist cakes and everything in between. Air fryers are popular because they can give the food the fried crispiness without frying them at all, which is healthier than any fried foods but equally delicious or more.

In around 2013, air fryers first entered the market and now have become the kitchens' sensation. They will offer a crisp outer shell to your favorite foods without submerging them in oil. Think about Healthier French fries; although these terms do not go together, it is possible now, and the reason is cooking in the air fryer. Cooking on a sheet pan will give an equal performance, but it turns out the air fryer is quick, simple, and handy. So when baking, roasting in the oven becomes too much work give your time to air fryer; they will not let you down. Cooking with Air fryer on every standard is easier than frying in oil. It decreases calories by 70-80% and has less fat. Any of the other adverse consequences of oil frying may also be minimized by this form of cooking. That eventually allows the appetite for fried food a cooler and healthier option. The potential of air fryers to cook and reheat leftovers is remarkable. Foods such as arancini egg rolls, and taquitos, look as amazing as they tasted when they are made fresh. So, let's get started with delicious healthy, and affordable air fryer recipes.

Chapter 1: Air Fryer Tips & Tricks

In the way, an air fryer roasts and bakes is identical to an oven. Still, the distinction is that the heating source is placed only on top and is assisted by a big, strong fan that spreads the heat equally, resulting in super crispy and healthy food in less time, and most importantly, with much less oil than deep frying equivalents. Usually, air fryers warm up very easily and, due to the fusion of a centralized heat source and a fan's placement, air fry cooks food uniformly and quickly.

The cleanup is yet another best part of the air fryer. Many racks and baskets of air fryers can be cleaned in the dishwasher. We recommend a decent dish brush for those who are not dishwasher safe. Without making oneself crazy, the soft bristle brush can get through all cracks and crevices that encourage air circulation to cook crispier food.

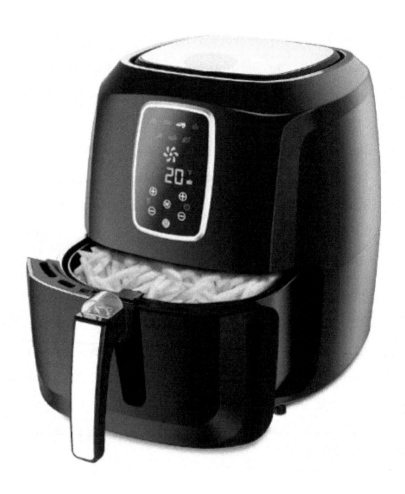

1.1 Air fryer Cheat Sheet

INGREDIENT	TEMP	TIME	PREP
CHICKEN BREASTS, 6 oz each	380°F	10 TO 15 MIN.	Brush with oil, season and flip halfway through cooking.
CHICKEN WINGS, split, 1 lb	400°F	20 TO 25 MIN.	Toss with seasoning.
CHICKEN THIGHS, bone-in	400°F	15 TO 20 MIN.	Season and arrange skin side up.
PORK CHOPS, bone-in, 1 in. thick	400°F	10 TO 15 MIN.	Season and flip halfway through cooking.
STEAK, 1 in. thick	400°F	10 TO 15 MIN.	Season and flip halfway through cooking.
FISH FILLETS, 1 in. thick, 6 oz each	400°F	8 TO 10 MIN.	Brush with oil and season.
SWEET POTATOES, cut into 1-in. wedges	400°F	12 TO 15 MIN.	Toss with oil, season and shake basket halfway through cooking.
BRUSSELS SPROUTS, halved	400°F	10 TO 15 MIN.	Toss with oil, season and shake basket twice during cooking.
BUTTERNUT SQUASH, cut into 1-in. pieces	400°F	12 TO 15 MIN.	Toss with oil, season and shake basket halfway through cooking.
FROZEN FRIES, 1 lb.	400°F	15 TO 20 MIN.	Shake twice during cooking.

1.2 Tips & Tricks

- Before loading the air fryer with food, you should always preheat the air fryer.
- Put a piece of bread in the air fryer's bottom so that it will catch fat from fatty foods without creating a mess.

- Choose the correct air fryer for your needs, so do your research beforehand.
- During air frying or roasting, shake the basket a couple of times to ensure it cooks uniformly.
- For a safety measure, spray the cooking food with oil only after taking the basket out completely.
- Reheat the leftovers in an air fryer rather than in the microwave; it will crisp them right up.
- Do not put too much food in the air fryer's basket; leave some room for the hot to circulate.
- Use less oil in air frying because less is more.
- Add water to the bottom drawer for fatty foods so that it will prevent smoking
- Clean the air fryer as one finishes using it.
- Using cookbooks for air fryers, like this one, to master the art of air frying.**1.3 Cooking Conversion Chart**

Use a cooking conversion chart for your ease

COOKING CONVERSION CHART

Measurement

CUP	ONCES	MILLILITERS	TABLESPOONS
8 cup	64 oz	1895 ml	128
6 cup	48 oz	1420 ml	96
5 cup	40 oz	1180 ml	80
4 cup	32 oz	960 ml	64
2 cup	16 oz	480 ml	32
1 cup	8 oz	240 ml	16
3/4 cup	6 oz	177 ml	12
2/3 cup	5 oz	158 ml	11
1/2 cup	4 oz	118 ml	8
3/8 cup	3 oz	90 ml	6
1/3 cup	2.5 oz	79 ml	5.5
1/4 cup	2 oz	59 ml	4
1/8 cup	1 oz	30 ml	3
1/16 cup	1/2 oz	15 ml	1

Temperature

FAHRENHEIT	CELSIUS
100 °F	37 °C
150 °F	65 °C
200 °F	93 °C
250 °F	121 °C
300 °F	150 °C
325 °F	160 °C
350 °F	180 °C
375 °F	190 °C
400 °F	200 °C
425 °F	220 °C
450 °F	230 °C
500 °F	260 °C
525 °F	274 °C
550 °F	286 °C

Weight

IMPERIAL	METRIC
1/2 oz	15 g
1 oz	29 g
2 oz	57 g
3 oz	85 g
4 oz	113 g
5 oz	141 g
6 oz	170 g
8 oz	227 g
10 oz	283 g
12 oz	340 g
13 oz	369 g
14 oz	397 g
15 oz	425 g
1 lb	453 g

Chapter 2: Air-Fryer Appetizers & Snacks

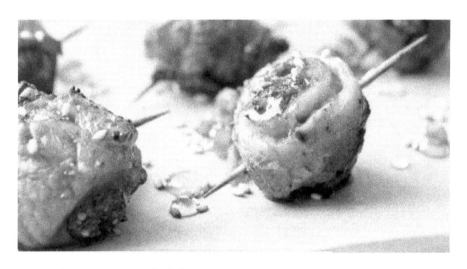

1. Air-Fryer Pickles

(Ready in about 30 minutes| Serving 32|Difficulty: Easy)

Nutrition per 1 slice of a pickle: Calories 26 |Carbs 4g|Protein 1g |Fat 3 g

Ingredients

- All-purpose flour: Half cup
- 2 tbsp. of dill pickle juice
- Dill pickle: 32 slices
- 3 eggs, lightly whisked
- Half tsp. Of cayenne pepper

- Panko bread crumbs: 2 cups
- Half tsp. of salt
- 2 tbsp. of chopped fresh dill
- Half tsp. of garlic powder

Instructions

- Let the air fryer preheat to 400 F. Dry the pickles well with a paper towel and let them rest on a paper towel for 15 minutes.
- In a bowl, mix salt and flour. In a separate bowl, beat the eggs with garlic powder, pickle juice, and cayenne.
- In another bowl, mix the dill and panko.
- Coat the pickles in the flour mix, then in egg mixture, then coat in panko mixture, pat them so coating with a stick.
- Oil spray the air fryer basket and place coated pickles in the basket in one even layer.
- Cook for 7 to 10 minutes, flip the pickles and spray with oil cook for another 7 to 10 minutes.
- Cook in batches and serve right away with your choice of dressing.

2. Sriracha Crispy Spring Rolls

(Ready in about 60 minutes| Serving 24|Difficulty: Medium)

Nutrition per serving: Calories 127 |Carbs 10 g| Protein 6g |Fat 7 g

Ingredients

- 3 green onions, diced
- Seasoned salt: 1 tsp.
- Soy sauce: 1 tbsp.
- Coleslaw mix: 3 cups
- Sriracha chili sauce: 2 tbsp.
- Sesame oil: 1 tsp.
- 1 pound of skinless chicken breasts (boneless)
- Spring roll wrappers: 24
- Softened cream cheese (8 oz. each): 2 packages

Instructions

- Let the air fryer preheat to 360 F.
- In a bowl, mix sesame oil, green onions, soy sauce, and coleslaw mix. Set it aside.
- Oil Spray the air fryer's basket, place chicken in the basket in one even layer, and cook for 18 to 20 minutes until internal chicken temperature reaches 165°.
- Take chicken out and let it cool for a bit. Dice the chicken and season with seasoned salt.
- Now, let the air fryer heat to 400 F.

- In a bowl, mix Sriracha sauce and cream cheese, add in coleslaw mixture and chicken.
- Place roll wrapper on a clean surface on one corner facing you, add 2 tbsp. of chicken filling more on the corner side.
- Fold the spring roll tightly and seal the edges with water.
- Place spring rolls in the oiled air fryer basket in one-layer cook for 5 to 6 minutes. Flip the rolls spray with oil, and cook for another 5 to 6 minutes.
- Serve right away with sweet chili sauce.

3. Buffalo Cauliflower Bites

(Ready in about 50 minutes| Serving 4|Difficulty: Medium)

Nutrition per serving: Calories 125 |Carbs 17 g| Protein 5 g |Fat 4 g

Ingredients

- Half head of (3-lb.) Cauliflower, slice into one-inch florets
- Hot sauce: 2 tbsp.
- Crumbled blue cheese: 1 tbsp.
- 1 egg white
- Sour cream, reduced-fat: 1/4 cup

- Panko: 3/4 cup
- Ketchup: 3 tbsp.
- Black pepper: 1/4 tsp.
- Red wine vinegar: 1 tsp.
- 1 minced clove of garlic

Instructions

- In a bowl, mix egg white with hot sauce and ketchup until it becomes smooth.

- In a bowl, add the panko. Coat the cauliflower pieces with ketchup mix.

- Now coat the cauliflower pieces in panko. Spray the cauliflower generously with oil spray.

- Add only half of the coated cauliflower in an oiled air fryer basket in one even layer.

- Roast for 20 minutes at 320 F until crispy and light brown.

- In the meantime, mix vinegar, sour cream, garlic, black pepper, and blue cheese. Mix well and serve with buffalo cauliflower.

4. Air-Fried Calzones

(Ready in about 27 minutes| Serving 2|Difficulty: Medium)

Nutrition per serving: Calories 348 |Carbs 44 g| Protein 21 g |Fat 12 g

Ingredients

- Baby spinach leaves: 3 cups
- Extra virgin olive oil: 1 tsp.
- 6 oz. of prepared pizza dough (whole-wheat)
- Finely diced red onion: 1/4 cup
- Shredded mozzarella cheese: 6 tbsp.
- Rotisserie shredded chicken breast: 1/3 cup
- Marinara sauce, low-sodium: 1/3 cup

Instructions

- In a cast-iron skillet, heat the oil and sauté onion for 2 minutes until tender.

- Add spinach, cover the skillet and cook until it wilts for about one and a half minutes. Turn off the heat, add in chicken and marinara sauce.

- Slice the dough into four portions. Roll each piece into a six" circle.

- Add 1/4th of the spinach mixture on the circled dough and add 1/4th of cheese on one half of the circle.

- Fold the other half over the filling and seal the edges and crimp them.

- Spray the calzones with oil spray.

- Put the calzones in an oiled air fryer basket. Cook for 12 minutes at 325 F until the dough is light brown. Flip the calzones and cook for 8 more minutes.

- Serve right.

5. Sweet Potato Tots

(Ready in about 1 hour & 20 minutes| Serving 4|Difficulty: Hard)

Nutrition per serving: Calories 78 |Carbs 19 g| Protein 1 g |Fat 0 g

Ingredients

- 1 and 1/4 tsp. of kosher salt, divided
- 2 small peeled sweet potatoes
- 1/8 tsp. of garlic powder
- 1 tbsp. of potato starch

- 3/4 cup of ketchup

Instructions

- In a pot, add water and let it boil on high flame. Boil potatoes for 15 minutes until fork tender.
- Take them out on a plate and let them cool for 15 minutes.
- Grate the potatoes in a bowl, and mix with 1 tsp. of salt, potato starch, and garlic powder.
- Make 24 tots like shapes from this grated potato mixture.
- Oil Spray the air fryer's basket. Put half of the tots in the basket in one even layer and spray them with oil spray.
- Cook for 12-14 minutes at 400°F until golden brown; flip them halfway through. Take out from air fryer and sprinkle with 1/8 tsp of salt and enjoy with ketchup.

6. Sweet Potato Chips

(Ready in about 40 minutes| Serving 4|Difficulty: Easy)

Nutrition per serving: Calories 357 |Carbs 28 g| Protein 2 g |Fat 27 g

Ingredients

- Ground Cinnamon: 1 tsp.
- 2 Sweet Potatoes, cut into thin slices
- Salt & black pepper, to taste
- Extra virgin Olive Oil: ¼ cup

Instructions

- In cold water, soak the thinly cut potatoes for half an hour.
- Discard the water and with paper dry the slices. Make them completely dry so they will get crispy.
- Coat the slices with olive oil, black pepper, cinnamon, and salt. Make sure every piece is coated with oil and seasoning.
- Oil Spray the air fryer's basket.
- Air fry the slices for 20 minutes at 390 F, shake the basket every 7 to 8 minutes.
- Cook for an additional five minutes if they are not crispy enough.
- Serve right away with a dipping sauce.

7. Churros with Chocolate Sauce

(Ready in about 1 hour & 25 minutes| Serving 12|Difficulty: Hard)

Nutrition per serving: Calories 173|Carbs 12 g| Protein 3 g |Fat 11 g

Ingredients

- Half cup of bittersweet chocolate, finely diced
- Half cup of water
- Unsalted butter: 1/4 cup + 2 tbsp.
- Kosher salt: 1/4 tsp.
- Heavy cream: 3 tbsp.
- 2 whole eggs
- Granulated sugar: 1/3 cup
- Half cup of all-purpose flour
- Vanilla kefir: 2 tbsp.
- Ground cinnamon: 2 tsp.

Instructions

- In a pot, add salt, ¼ cup of butter, and water. Let it boil over medium flame.
- Turn the heat to low add flour with a wooden spoon mix vigorously for 30 seconds until dough becomes smooth.
- Keep stirring, for 2-3 minutes, until the dough starts to pull away from the pot.

- Take the dough out in a bowl. Slightly cool it by constantly stirring for one minute.

- Add the eggs, one by one, keep stirring until the dough becomes completely smooth.

- Place the mixture in the piping bag with a medium tip. Chill for half an hour.

- Place six pieces (three" long) of piped dough in one even layer in an oiled air fryer basket.

- Air fry for ten minutes, at 380°F.

- In a bowl, mix cinnamon and sugar. Coat the churros in 2 tbsp. of melted butter and coat in the sugar mix.

- In a microwave-safe bowl, add cream and chocolate. Microwave for 30 seconds mix after 15 seconds. Add in kefir and serve with churros.

8. Rosemary & Garlic Brussels Sprouts

(Ready in about 30 minutes| Serving 4|Difficulty: Easy)

Nutrition per serving: Calories 164|Carbs 15 g| Protein 5 g |Fat 11 g

Ingredients

- Panko bread crumbs: half cup

- Olive oil: 3 tbsp.
- Half tsp. Of salt
- Chopped fresh rosemary: 1 and a half tsp.
- Black Pepper: 1/4 tsp.
- 1 pound of Brussels sprouts, cleaned & cut in halves
- 2 minced cloves of garlic

Instructions

- Let the air fryer preheat to 350 F.
- Add olive oil, minced garlic, black pepper, and salt— microwave for 30 seconds on high.
- Coat Brussels sprouts with 2 tbsp. of the oil mix.
- Oil Spray the air fryer's basket, put Brussel sprouts in the basket, and cook for five minutes.
- Stir the basket. Cook for 8 more minutes, until tender and crispy. Again, stir the basket halfway through cooking.
- In a bowl, mix the rest of the oil mixture with rosemary and crumbs. Sprinkle the bread crumbs over Brussel sprouts. Cook for 3 to 5 minutes.
- Serve right away.

9. Pumpkin Fries

(Ready in about 40 minutes| Serving 4|Difficulty: Easy)

Nutrition per serving: Calories 151|Carbs 31 g| Protein 5 g |Fat 3 g

Ingredients

- Chipotle peppers in adobo sauce: 2-3 tsp. (minced)
- Garlic powder: 1/4 tsp.
- Half cup Greek yogurt (plain)
- Maple syrup: 2 tbsp.
- 1/8 tsp. + half tsp. Salt
- Black pepper: 1/4 tsp.
- Chili powder: 1/4 tsp.
- 1 pie pumpkin (medium)
- Ground cumin: 1/4 tsp.

Instructions

- In a bowl, mix chipotle peppers, yogurt, 1/8 tsp. of salt, and maple syrup. Mix and keep in the fridge covered.
- Let the air fryer preheat to 400 F.
- Peel and slice the pumpkin in half. Take out the seeds.
- Slice into half-inch of strips and add to a bowl.
- Sprinkle with half tsp. of salt, chili powder, cumin, pepper, and garlic powder, coat well.
- Oil Spray the air fryer's basket. Place pumpkin fries in the basket.

- Cook for 6 to 8 minutes until tender. Stir the basket and cook for 3 to 5 minutes more until light brown.
- Serve with prepared dipping sauce.

10. Loaded Potatoes

(Ready in about 25 minutes| Serving 2-3|Difficulty: Medium)

Nutrition per serving: Calories 199|Carbs 26 g| Protein 7 g |Fat 7 g

Ingredients

- Sour cream, reduced-fat: 2 tbsp.
- 8 baby Yukon gold potatoes
- Olive oil: 1 tsp.
- 2 slices of bacon (center-cut)
- Kosher salt: 1/8 tsp.
- Shredded cheddar cheese, reduced-fat: 2 tbsp.
- Chopped fresh chives: 1 and a half tbsp.

Instructions

- Coat the potatoes in olive oil. Put potatoes in the air fryer basket and cook for 25 minutes at 350 F; keep stirring the basket after every 5-8 minutes.
- In a skillet, cook the bacon for 7 minutes, at medium flame, until it becomes crispy.

- Take out from the pan and crumble the bacon.
- Take potatoes out on a serving plate and slightly crush them.
- Pour bacon fat over them. Serve with salt, bacon, sour cream, and chives on top.

11. Avocado Fries

(Ready in about 20 minutes| Serving 4|Difficulty: Easy)

Nutrition per serving: Calories 178|Carbs 18 g| Protein 12 g |Fat 2 g

Ingredients

- One can of garbanzo beans (15 oz.): aquafaba only
- Half cup of panko breadcrumbs
- One avocado, pitted & sliced
- Half tsp. of salt

Instructions

- In a bowl, mix the salt and panko.
- Pour the garbanzo liquid (aquafaba) into another bowl.
- Coat the avocado slices in aquafaba, then in bread crumbs mix, coat the slices well.
- Place the breaded slices in the basket of air fryer in one even layer.

- Air fry for ten minutes. Shake the basket after five minutes.
- Serve and enjoy.

12. Crispy French Fries

(Ready in about 30 minutes| Serving 4|Difficulty: Easy)

Nutrition per serving: Calories 189|Carbs 17 g| Protein 9 g |Fat 5 g

Ingredients

- Salt, to taste
- 3 russet potatoes
- Chopped fresh parsley: 2 tbsp.
- Olive oil: 1 tbsp.
- Parmesan cheese: 2 tbsp.

Instructions

- Slice the potatoes into French fries.
- With the paper towel, dry them completely.
- In a bowl, mix olive oil, cheese, parsley, and salt. Coat the French fries in this seasoning mix.
- Let the air fryer preheat to 360 F. Oil Spray the air fryer's basket.
- Place French fries in the basket in one even layer— Cook for 10 minutes.

- Stir the basket after ten minutes. Cook for 10 minutes more.
- Serve with dipping sauce and enjoy.

13. Spanakopita Morsels

(Ready in about 45 minutes| Serving 8|Difficulty: Medium)

Nutrition per serving: Calories 82|Carbs 7 g| Protein 4 g |Fat 4 g

Ingredients

- Water: 2 tbsp.
- 1 package of baby spinach leaves (10-oz.)
- Kosher salt: 1/4 tsp.
- Black pepper: 1/4 tsp.
- Feta cheese, crumbled: 1/4 cup
- 1 egg white
- Cottage cheese, low-fat: 1/4 cup
- Grated parmesan cheese: 2 tbsp.
- Lemon zest: 1 tsp.
- Dried oregano: 1 tsp.
- Olive oil: 1 tbsp.
- 4 sheets of phyllo dough
- Cayenne pepper: 1/8 tsp.

Instructions

- In a pot, add water and spinach and cook for five minutes until it wilts.
- Drain the water and let it cool for ten minutes. Squeeze out as much moister as possible.
- In a bowl, mix egg white, spinach, feta cheese, oregano, cayenne pepper, Parmesan cheese, black pepper, salt, and zest. Mix it well.
- Place one dough sheet on a clean surface. Spray with oil, and add a second layer of dough on top of it. Spray with oil. Keep adding layers all four layers.
- Slice the layers into 8 pieces. Slice in further half so you will get 16 pieces.
- Add one tbsp. of filling in one piece of phyllo. Fold it in a triangle.
- Oil spray the air fryer's basket. Place the 8 phyllo bites in one even layer in the basket, spray with oil.
- Cook for 12 minutes at 375 F, until golden brown. Flip the bites halfway through.

- Serve right away.

14. Sweet & Spicy Meatballs

(Ready in about 40 minutes| Serving 15|Difficulty: Medium)

Nutrition per serving: Calories 90|Carbs 10 g| Protein 6 g |Fat 3 g

Ingredients

- 2 pounds of lean ground beef
- Crushed Ritz crackers: Half cup
- 2 eggs, lightly whisked
- Quick-cooking oats: 2/3 cup
- Salt: 1 tsp.
- 1 can of (5 oz.) Evaporated milk
- Honey: 1 tsp.
- Garlic powder: 1 tsp.
- Half tsp. of pepper
- Dried minced onion: 1 tbsp.
- Ground cumin: 1 tsp.

Sauce

- 1 tbsp. of Worcestershire sauce
- Packed brown sugar: 1/3 cup
- 1-2 tbsp. of Louisiana-style hot sauce
- orange marmalade: 1/3 cup
- 2 tbsp. of cornstarch
- Honey: 1/3 cup
- 2 tbsp. of soy sauce

Instructions

- Let the air fryer preheat to 380 F.
- In a bowl, add all the meatballs ingredients. Mix it well.
- Make one-and-a-half-inch meatballs.
- Oil spray the air fryer's basket—place meatballs in the basket in one even layer.
- Cook for 12 to 15 minutes, until cooked through.
- In a small bowl, add all the sauce ingredients. Cook on medium flame until thickens.
- Serve meatballs with sauce.

15. Crispy Onion Rings with Sauce

(Ready in about 55 minutes| Serving 4|Difficulty: Medium)

Nutrition per serving: Calories 174|Carbs 25 g| Protein 7 g |Fat 5 g

Ingredients

- Smoked paprika: 1 tsp.
- Ketchup: 1 tbsp.
- Half cup of all-purpose flour
- Water: 1 tbsp.
- 1 egg
- 1/4 tsp. of paprika

- 1/4 tsp. of garlic powder
- 1 sweet onion, slice into 1/2-inch-thick circles & separated
- Whole-wheat panko: 1 cup
- Canola mayonnaise: 2 tbsp.
- Dijon mustard: 1 tsp.
- Low-fat Greek yogurt: 1/4 cup
- Half tsp. of kosher salt

Instructions

- In a dish, mix the smoked paprika,1/4 tsp. salt, flour.
- In a bowl, whisk the egg with water.
- In a separate bowl, mix the panko with ¼ tsp. salt.
- Coat onions in flour mix then in the egg mixture. Coat in the panko mixture.
- Spray the breaded onion rings with oil spray.
- Put onion rings in the basket of the air fryer in one single layer—Cook for ten minutes at 375 F.
- Flip the onion rings halfway through—Cook the remaining onion rings.
- In a bowl, mix garlic powder, yogurt, ketchup, paprika, mayonnaise, and mustard.
- Serve the onion rings with sauce.

16. Crunchy Corn Dog Bites

(Ready in about 35 minutes| Serving 4|Difficulty: Medium)

Nutrition per serving: Calories 82|Carbs 8 g| Protein 5 g |Fat 3 g

Ingredients

- Yellow mustard: 8 tsp.
- 2 beef hot dogs uncured
- 1 and a half cups of crushed cornflakes
- Half cup of all-purpose flour
- Bamboo skewers: 12
- 2 eggs, lightly whisked

Instructions

- Cut hot dogs in halves. Slice every half into three pieces.
- Thread them on bamboo skewers.
- Add flour to a dish. Add eggs to another dish.
- Add cornflakes to another dish.
- Coat the hot dogs in flour, then in egg, and then coat in crushed corn flakes.
- Oil spray the air fryer's basket. Put hot dog skewers in the basket in one even layer.

- Cook for ten minutes at 375 F until crunchy and brown. Flip them halfway through cooking.
- Serve with mustard.

17. Ranch Kale Chips

(Ready in about 12 minutes| Serving 2|Difficulty: Easy)

Nutrition per serving: Calories 82|Carbs 8 g| Protein 5 g |Fat 3 g

Ingredients

- Salt, a pinch
- Loosely packed kale: 4 cups remove stems
- Any seasoning mix: 1 to 2 tbsp.
- Olive oil: 2 tsp.

Instructions

- Coat the kale with olive oil and salt.
- Place the kale in the air fryer basket.
- Cook for 4 to 6 minutes at 370 F. (No need to preheat).
- Stir the basket every two minutes. Keep checking for your desired doneness.
- Sprinkle with seasoning of your choice and serve right away.

18. Cheese Sticks

(Ready in about 22 minutes| Serving 6|Difficulty: Easy)

Nutrition per serving: Calories 67|Carbs 5 g| Protein 5 g |Fat 3 g

Ingredients

- 6 medium-sized cheese sticks
- 1/4 tsp. ground rosemary
- 2 whole eggs
- Grated parmesan cheese: 1/4 cup
- Garlic powder: 1 tsp.
- Whole wheat flour: 1/4 cup
- Italian Seasoning: 1 tsp.

Instructions

- In a bowl, whisk the eggs well.
- In a separate bowl, mix the cheese, flour, and seasoning.
- Coat the cheese sticks in eggs, then in the flour mix. Coat them well.
- Place the breaded cheese sticks in an air fryer in a single even layer.
- Cook for 6 to 7 minutes at 370 F.
- Serve with marinara sauce and enjoy.

19. Cinnamon-Dusted Apple Chips

(Ready in about 20 minutes| Serving 8|Difficulty: Easy)

Nutrition per serving: Calories 178|Carbs 39 g| Protein 1 g |Fat 1 g

Ingredients

- Avocado Oil: 1 tbsp.
- 6 Apples
- Cinnamon: 1 tbsp.

Instructions

- With a mandolin, cut the apples into thin slices.
- Coat the apple slices with avocado oil and sprinkle with cinnamon.
- Let the air fryer preheat to 400 F.
- Cook the apple chips at 400 F for 15 minutes.
- Serve and enjoy.

20. Crispy Vegetable Quesadillas

(Ready in about 40 minutes| Serving 4|Difficulty: Medium)

Nutrition per serving: Calories 291|Carbs 36 g| Protein 17 g |Fat 8 g

Ingredients

- Canned black beans: 1 cup, drained & rinsed
- Red bell pepper, sliced: 1 cup
- Sharp cheddar cheese, shredded: 1 cup
- Chopped fresh cilantro: 2 tbsp.
- Greek yogurt, reduced-fat: 4 tbsp.
- 1 tsp. Lime zest + 1 tbsp. of lime juice
- Half cup drained Pico de Gallo
- 4 whole flour tortillas, (six-inch)
- Ground cumin: 1/4 tsp.
- Sliced zucchini: 1 cup

Instructions

- Put tortillas on a clean surface. Add 2 tbsp. of shredded cheese on half of the tortilla.
- Add black beans, 1/4 cup of pepper slices, zucchini slices, and a half cup of cheese.
- Fold the tortilla overfilling. Coat with cooking spray and close with toothpicks if necessary.
- Oil spray the air fryer's basket. Place 2 quesadillas in the air fryer.
- Cook for ten minutes at 400 F, until cheese is melted and it is golden brown.
- In a bowl, mix lime juice, yogurt, cumin, and lime zest.

- Slice and serve the quesadilla with yogurt sauce and Pico de Gallo.

21. Greek Loaded Feta Fries

(Ready in about 45 minutes| Serving 2|Difficulty: Medium)

Nutrition per serving: Calories 383|Carbs 42 g| Protein 19 g |Fat 16 g

Ingredients

- 2 russet potatoes, cleaned & dried
- Half cup of rotisserie chicken breast, shredded (skinless)
- Garlic powder: 1/4 tsp.
- Olive oil: 1 tbsp.
- Half tsp. of dried oregano
- Lemon zest: 2 tsp.
- Onion powder: 1/4 tsp.
- Kosher salt: 1/4 tsp.
- Chopped red onion: 2 tbsp.
- Black pepper: 1/4 tsp.
- Feta cheese, crumbled: half cup
- Prepared tzatziki: 1/4 cup
- Paprika: 1/4 tsp.
- Chopped fresh oregano & parsley: 1 tbsp.

- Plum tomato, diced: 1/4 cup

Instructions

- Let the air fryer preheat to 380 F. Oil spray the air fryer's basket.
- Slice the potatoes in half and cut into ¼" thick slices, then cut into fries.
- Toss the potatoes with oil and onion powder, zest, pepper, garlic powder, dried oregano, paprika, and salt.
- Place the half of fries in the air fryer basket in one even layer and cook for 15 minutes; stir the basket halfway through.
- Serve fries with red onion, chicken, feta, tzatziki, fresh herbs on top.

22. Pepper Poppers

(Ready in about 35 minutes| Serving 2 dozen| Difficulty: Medium)

Nutrition one pepper: Calories 81|Carbs 18 g| Protein 3 g |Fat 6 g

Ingredients

- Half cup of dry bread crumbs
- Cheddar cheese, shredded: 3/4 cup

- Shredded Monterey Jack cheese: 3/4 cup
- Garlic powder: 1/4 tsp.
- 1 package of softened cream cheese (8 oz.)
- 6 strips of bacon, cooked & crumbled
- Salt: 1/4 tsp.
- Smoked paprika: 1/4 tsp.
- 1 pound of jalapenos (fresh), cut into halves and remove seeds
- Chili powder: 1/4 tsp.

Instructions

- Let the air fryer preheat to 325 F.
- In a bowl, mix seasonings, cheese, and bacon.
- Add almost 2 tbsp. of filling in every half of the pepper. Coat in bread crumbs.
- Oil spray the air fryer's basket—place peppers in the basket in one even layer.
- Cook for 15 to 20 minutes, or until cheese is melted.
- Serve with your favorite dipping sauce.

23. Wasabi Crab Cakes

(Ready in about 30 minutes| Serving 2 dozen| Difficulty: Medium)

Nutrition per serving: Calories 49|Carbs 4 g| Protein 3 g |Fat 2 g

Ingredients

- 1 and a half cups of lump crabmeat
- 1 sweet red pepper, finely diced
- 3 chopped green onions
- Wasabi: 1/4 tsp.
- 2 egg whites
- 1 diced celery rib
- 1/3 cup + half cup of dry bread crumbs
- 3 tbsp. of mayonnaise reduced-fat
- Salt: 1/4 tsp.

Sauce

- Half tsp. of prepared wasabi
- Sweet pickle relish: 1 tbsp.
- 1 diced celery rib
- Celery salt: 1/4 tsp.
- Reduced-fat mayonnaise: 1/3 cup
- 1 chopped green onion

Instructions

- Let the air fryer preheat to 375 F.

- Add all ingredients except for sauce, bread crumbs, and crab meat; only add 1/3 cup of bread crumbs. Carefully fold in the crab meat.
- Add the rest of the bread crumbs in a bowl. Makes ¾ "patties of crab meat and coat in bread crumbs.
- Oil spray the air fryer's basket.
- Place the patties into the basket, and cook for 8 to 12 minutes.
- Flip them halfway through cooking, spray with cooking oil, and cook.
- In a food processor place all sauce ingredients, pulse to reach desired texture and serve with crab cakes.

24. Mini Burritos

(Ready in about 40 minutes| Serving 2 | Difficulty: Medium)

Nutrition per serving: Calories 121|Carbs 5 g| Protein 8 g |Fat 3 g

Ingredients

- 4 pieces of rice paper
- Cashew butter: 2 tbsp.
- Tamari: 2 to 3 tbsp.

- Liquid smoke: 1 to 2 tbsp.

- Tofu Scramble, as needed

- 1 to 2 tbsp. of water

Vegetables

- 1 sautéed small tree of broccoli

- Sweet potato cubes, roasted: 1/3 cup

- Handful of kale, or spinach

- 8 strips of red pepper, roasted

- 6 to 8 stalks of fresh asparagus

Instructions

- Let the air fryer preheat to 350 F.
- Mix all the ingredients in a bowl except for rice paper.
- Place filling in the rice paper, and spray with cooking oil.
- Oil spray the air fryer's basket.
- Place the rolls in the basket and cook for 8 to 10 minutes until crispy.

25. Caribbean Wontons

(Ready in about 40 minutes| Serving 2 dozen| Difficulty: Medium)

Nutrition per serving: Calories 83|Carbs 13 g| Protein 1 g |Fat 3 g

Ingredients

- Wonton wrappers: 24
- Softened cream cheese: half cup
- Marshmallow crème: 1 cup
- Mashed ripe banana: 1/4 cup
- Chopped walnuts: 2 tbsp.
- Sweetened coconut, shredded: 1/4 cup
- Crushed pineapple, canned: 2 tbsp.

Sauce

- Ground cinnamon & Confectioners' sugar, as needed
- Fresh strawberries halves: 1 pound
- Cornstarch: 1 tsp.
- Sugar: 1/4 cup

Instructions

- Let the air fryer preheat to 350 F.
- In a bowl, beat the cream cheese. Add in pineapple, coconut, walnuts, and bananas. Add in marshmallow crème.
- On a clean surface lay a piece of wonton, one edge facing towards you.

- Add 2 tsp. of filling in the middle of the wrapper. Seal the edges with water and fold the corners facing each other.
- Fill in all the wontons like this.
- Oil spray the air fryer's basket and place wonton in the basket in one even layer and spray with cooking oil.
- Cook at 350 F for 10 to 12 minutes.
- In a food processor, add strawberries and make a puree.
- In a small pot, mix cornstarch and sugar add in strawberry puree. Let it boil for 2 minutes until it thickens.
- Strain the sauce if you like otherwise, serve it as it is with wontons, dusted with cinnamon and confectioners' sugar.

26. Curry Chickpeas

(Ready in about 25 minutes| Serving 4| Difficulty: Easy)

Nutrition per serving: Calories 173|Carbs 18 g| Protein 7 g |Fat 8 g

Ingredients

- 1/4 tsp. of ground cumin

- 1 can of (15-oz.) chickpeas no-salt-added, drained & rinsed
- 2 tsp. of curry powder
- Half tsp. of Aleppo pepper
- 2 tbsp. of red wine vinegar
- Half tsp. of ground turmeric
- 1/4 tsp. of ground coriander
- Fresh cilantro, chopped
- 1/4 tsp. + 1/8 tsp. of ground cinnamon
- 2 tbsp. of olive oil
- 1/4 tsp. kosher salt

Instructions

- Carefully lightly smash the chickpeas with clean hands in a bowl, and discard the skin but do not crush chickpeas.
- Mix the chickpeas with oil, vinegar. Add cinnamon, curry powder, cumin, coriander, and turmeric toss well.
- Add chickpeas in one even layer to an oiled air fryer basket and cook at 400 F for 15 minutes, until crispy; shake the basket halfway through.
- Take chickpeas out in the bowl—season with Aleppo pepper, salt. Top with cilantro and serve.

27. Shrimp Spring Rolls with Sweet Chili Sauce

(Ready in about 35 minutes| Serving 4| Difficulty: Medium)

Nutrition per serving: Calories 180|Carbs 19 g| Protein 7 g |Fat 9 g

Ingredients

- 8 spring roll wrappers, (8"-square)
- Pre-shredded cabbage: 2 cups
- Matchstick carrots: 1 cup
- 2 and a half tbsp. of sesame oil
- 4 ounces of peeled, deveined uncooked shrimp, diced
- Red bell pepper, julienne-cut: 1 cup
- Fresh cilantro, chopped: 1/4 cup
- Half cup of sweet chili sauce
- 1 tbsp. of fresh lime juice
- 2 tsp. of fish sauce
- 1/4 tsp. of crushed red pepper
- Julienne-cut snow peas: 3/4 cup

Instructions

- In a skillet, heat one and a half tsp. of oil, heat until it smokes. Add bell pepper, cabbage, and carrots. Keep stirring for 1 to one and a half minutes, until they lightly wilt.

- Take them out on a baking sheet and let them cool for five minutes.
- In a bowl, mix vegetable mix with snow peas, fish sauce, crushed red pepper, shrimp, lime juice, and cilantro. Toss well.
- On a clean work, surface lay one spring roll, one corner towards you. Add ¼ cup of filling on a spring roll. Place as three" long filling.
- Fold the wrapper over filling, seal the ends with water, and press.
- Brush all the rolls with 2 tbsp. of oil.
- Put rolls in the basket of air fryer and cook for 6-7 minutes at 390 F. flip the rolls after five minutes.
- Serve with sauce.

28. Peanut Chicken Egg Thai Rolls

(Ready in about 20 minutes| Serving 2| Difficulty: Easy)

Nutrition per serving: Calories 235|Carbs 17 g| Protein 7 g |Fat 7 g

Ingredients

- 1 carrot, cut into thin slices

- egg roll wrappers: 4
- 1/4 red bell pepper, cut into julienne style
- Thai peanut sauce: 1/4 cup
- 3 green onions, diced
- 2 cups of shredded rotisserie chicken

Instructions

- Let the air fryer preheat to 390 F
- In a bowl, mix shredded chicken with peanut sauce.
- On a surface, place one egg roll wrapper, and on the bottom, place thinly cut vegetables with half tsp. of chicken mix.
- Fold the wrapper tightly and seal the edges with water.
- Repeat the process with all the wrappers.
- Spray the egg rolls with oil spray on all sides.
- Put rolls in one layer in the air fryer and bake for 6 to 8 minutes at 390 F until crispy.
- Serve with dipping sauce and enjoy.

29. Tortellini with Prosciutto

(Ready in about 35 minutes| Serving 12| Difficulty: Medium)

Nutrition per serving: Calories 38|Carbs 5 g| Protein 1 g |Fat 1 g

Ingredients

- 1 can of (15 oz.) tomato puree
- Olive oil: 1 tbsp.
- 4 chopped cloves of garlic
- 1/4 tsp. black pepper
- Chopped fresh basil: 1 tbsp.
- Finely chopped onion: 3 tbsp.
- 1/4 tsp. salt

Tortellini

- 1 pack of (12 oz.) prosciutto ricotta tortellini
- 2 whole eggs
- Bread crumbs, seasoned: 2/3 cup
- Half tsp. of salt
- Garlic powder: 1 tsp.
- Pecorino cheese, grated: 2 tbsp.
- 2% milk: 2 tbsp.
- Fresh parsley, chopped: 1 tbsp.

Instructions

- In a pan, add oil over medium flame. Sauté garlic and onion for 3 to 4 minutes until tender. Add black pepper, tomato puree, salt, and basil.

- Let it boil, turn the heat low, and let it simmer for ten minutes. Do not cover the pot.
- Let the air fryer preheat to 350 F.
- In a bowl, mix milk and eggs.
- In a separate bowl, mix bread crumbs, salt, cheese, parsley, and garlic powder.
- Coat the tortellini in egg mix, secondly coat in crumb mix.
- Place tortellini in an oiled basket of air fryer in one even layer.
- Cook for 4 to 5 minutes, flip them spray with cooking spray, and coo =k for 4 to 5 minutes more.
- Top with chopped fresh basil and serve.

30. Rosemary Sausage Meatballs

(Ready in about 30 minutes| Serving 12| Difficulty: Medium)

Nutrition per serving: Calories 96|Carbs 2 g| Protein 4 g |Fat 8 g

Ingredients

- 2 tbsp. olive oil
- 2 pounds of pork sausage (bulk)
- 4 minced cloves of garlic

- Chopped fresh parsley: 1/4 cup
- 1 tsp. Curry powder
- 1 jar of (4 oz.) Chopped pimientos, drained
- 1 tbsp. Fresh rosemary, minced
- Dry bread crumbs: 1/4 cup
- 1 whole egg, lightly whisked

Instructions

- Let the air fryer preheat to 400 F.
- In a skillet, add oil over medium flame, sauté curry powder, and garlic for 1 to 2 minutes until tender. Let it cool slightly.
- In a mixing bowl, mix rosemary, egg, garlic mix, bread crumbs, parsley, and pimientos. Add sausage, mix well but do not over mix.
- Make into 1 or 1 and 1/4 "balls.
- Put in the basket of air fryer in one even layer, cook for 7 to 10 minutes until cooked through.
- Serve with sauce.

31. Buffalo Mushroom Poppers

(Ready in about 50 minutes| Serving 8| Difficulty: Medium)

Nutrition per serving: Calories 133|Carbs 16 g| Protein 7 g |Fat 4 g

Ingredients

- Apple cider vinegar: 3 tbsp.
- 1 pound of button mushrooms
- Buffalo hot sauce: 1/4 cup
- 1 jalapeño pepper, chopped without seeds
- 1 cup of panko
- Half tsp. kosher salt
- 2 whole eggs, lightly whisked
- 1/4 tsp. black pepper
- Less fat softened cream cheese: 3 tbsp.
- Half cup of crumbled blue cheese
- Half cup of buttermilk
- 1/4 cup of all-purpose flour
- Half cup of plain yogurt
- Chopped fresh chives: 2 tbsp.

Instructions

- Cut the stems of mushrooms, and chop them finely. Let the caps and stems aside.
- In a bowl, mix cream cheese, salt, mushroom stems, pepper, jalapenos, and salt.

- Place 1 tsp. of this mix into the caps of mushroom, make it a ball by rounding the stem filling.
- In a bowl, add panko. In another bowl, add flour, and in a separate bowl, add the eggs.
- Dip the mushroom balls in flour, then coat in egg, and lastly coat in panko mix.
- Spray the breaded mushroom with oil.
- Place these balls in one even layer in the basket of the air fryer.
- Cook for 20 minutes at 350 F, until crispy.
- Drizzle the cooked mushrooms with buffalo sauce. Serve with sauce and chives on top.
- In a bowl, mix blue cheese, cider vinegar, buttermilk, and yogurt. Serve the sauce with mushroom.

32. Turkey Croquettes

(Ready in about 30 minutes| Serving 6| Difficulty: Medium)

Nutrition per serving: Calories 322|Carbs 22 g| Protein 29 g |Fat 12 g

Ingredients

- Half cup of Parmesan cheese, grated

- Mashed potatoes: 2 cups (with milk & butter)
- 2 tbsp. Water
- 1 onion, finely diced
- Fresh rosemary, minced: 2 tsp.
- 1/4 tsp. of pepper
- Half cup of Swiss cheese, shredded
- Fresh sage, minced: 1 tsp.
- Half tsp. of salt
- 1 and 1/4 cups of panko bread crumbs
- 1 whole egg
- Diced cooked turkey: 3 cups

Instructions

- Let the air fryer preheat to 350 F.
- In a bowl, mix turkey, onion, cheese, mashed potato, pepper, rosemary, salt and sage.
- Make into one" thick 12 patties.
- In a bowl, mix water with egg. Add crumbs to another bowl.
- Coat patties in egg mix then in crumbs, coat them well.
- Place patties in one even layer in an oiled basket of air fryer, and spray the croquettes with cooking oil.
- Cook for 4 to 5 minutes, until golden brown.

- Flip the croquettes and spray with cooking oil—Cook for 4 to 5 more minutes.
- Serve right away and enjoy.

33. Beefy Swiss Bundles

(Ready in about 30 minutes| Serving 4| Difficulty: Medium)

Nutrition per serving: Calories 706|Carbs 44 g| Protein 35 g |Fat 42 g

Ingredients

- 1 and a half cups of sliced mushrooms
- 1 and a half tsp. of minced garlic
- 4 tsp. of Worcestershire sauce
- 1 sheet of puff pastry
- Half tsp. of salt
- Half cup of diced onion
- 1 pound of ground beef
- 3/4 tsp. of dried rosemary
- 3/4 tsp. of paprika
- 1 cup of shredded Swiss cheese
- 1/4 tsp. of pepper
- 2 tbsp. of water
- 2/3 cup of mashed potatoes, refrigerated

- 1 whole egg

Instructions

- Let the air fryer preheat to 375 F.
- In a skillet, cook mushrooms, beef, and onions on medium flame for 8 to 10 minutes, till beef is no longer pink.
- Add garlic and cook for 60 seconds more. Drain it and add seasonings and Worcestershire sauce.
- Roll dough in a rectangle (15 by 13"). Slice into four equal rectangles.
- Add 2 tbsp. of potatoes in every rectangle, spread it around. Add ¾ cup of beef mix and ¼ cup of cheese.
- In a small cup mix water with egg and brush over edges of puff pastry.
- Meet the opposite corners with each other and seal the edges.
- Brush the outer of pastry and place in air fryer's basket in one even layer and cook for 10 to 12 minutes, until light brown.

34. Cauliflower Gnocchi

(Ready in about 20 minutes| Serving 4| Difficulty: Easy)

Nutrition per serving: Calories 121|Carbs 4 g| Protein 3 g |Fat 4 g

Ingredients

- 1 pack of cauliflower gnocchi
- Sweet chili sauce, for serving

Instructions

- Let the air fryer preheat to 400 F.
- Oil spray the air fryer's basket.
- Make sure to thaw the gnocchi if using frozen.
- Spray with cooking spray and place in the air fryer, and cook for 20 minutes until crispy.
- Serve with sweet chili sauce.

35. Zucchini Chips

(Ready in about 20 minutes| Serving 4| Difficulty: Easy)

Nutrition per serving: Calories 130|Carbs 19 g| Protein 19 g |Fat 7 g

Ingredients

- ¼ cup of all-purpose flour
- 2 medium zucchinis
- Half cup of breadcrumbs
- 2 whole eggs

Instructions

- Cut the zucchini into ¼ inch thick slices.
- In three different bowls, add flour, bread crumbs, and whisked egg separately.
- Coat the zucchini coins in flour, then in whisked egg, and lastly coat in bread crumbs.
- Coat them again or three times, if required.
- Let the air fryer preheat to 355 F.
- Oil spray the air fryer's basket and place zucchini chips in one even layer in the basket.
- Cook for 4 minutes, flip and cook for 4 minutes more.
- Serve right away and enjoy.

36. Air-Fryer Taquitos

(Ready in about 35 minutes| Serving 10| Difficulty: Medium)

Nutrition per serving: Calories 168|Carbs 17g| Protein 12 g |Fat 6 g

Ingredients

- 1 pound of lean ground beef
- 2 whole eggs
- Taco seasoning: 3 tbsp.
- Corn tortillas: 10 pieces (6"), warmed

- Salsa & guacamole: optional
- Half cup dry bread crumbs

Instructions

- Let the air fryer preheat to 350 F.
- In a bowl, mix taco seasoning, bread crumbs, and eggs. Add beef and mix lightly.
- In every tortilla, place ¼ cup of the beef mixture and roll them tightly, secure with toothpicks if needed.
- Oil spray the air fryer's basket and place taquitos in one even layer.
- Cook at 350 F for 6 minutes, rotate them and cook for 6 to 7 minutes more, or until meat is completely cooked.
- Serve with guacamole & salsa.

37. Tortilla Chips

(Ready in about 20 minutes| Serving 2| Difficulty: Easy)

Nutrition per serving: Calories 373|Carbs 64 g| Protein 8 g |Fat 10 g

Ingredients

- Jazzy Spice Blend: 1 tbsp.
- 12 corn tortillas
- Kosher salt: 2 tsp.

- Olive oil: 1 tbsp.

Instructions

- Let the air fryer preheat to 350 F.
- With oil, brush the tortillas, covering every side.
- Season with spice blend and salt.
- Slice every tortilla into six wedges
- Place tortillas chips in an air fryer basket in one even layer and fry for five minutes.
- They should be crispy and light brown.
- Serve with salsa and guacamole.

38. Bacon-Wrapped Jalapeño Poppers

(Ready in about 30 minutes| Serving 9| Difficulty: Medium)

Nutrition per serving: Calories 256|Carbs 1 g| Protein 15 g |Fat 20 g

Ingredients

- Sharp cheddar cheese, shredded: ¾ cup
- 7 jalapeños, large
- ½ tsp. of kosher salt
- 14 strips of bacon
- 6 ounces of cream cheese softened

- ¼ tsp. of black pepper

Instructions

- Let the air fryer preheat to 325 F.
- Cut the jalapenos in half and remove membranes and seeds.
- In a bowl, mix cheddar cheese, pepper, cream cheese, and salt.
- Put the cheese mix in a piping bag with a small tip.
- Put the cheese mix into each half of jalapeno pepper.
- With one bacon strip, wrap the pepper.
- Place the pepper in the air fryer basket in one even layer and fry until bacon becomes crispy, for 8 to 10 minutes
- Serve right away and enjoy.

39. Eggplant Parmesan

(Ready in about 40 minutes| Serving 4| Difficulty: Easy)

Nutrition per serving: Calories 193|Carbs 5 g| Protein 11 g |Fat 8 g

Ingredients

- Marinara sauce: 1 cup
- 1 eggplant
- Salt, to taste

- Grated mozzarella cheese: 1/4 cup
- Whole wheat bread crumbs: half cup
- Italian seasoning mix: 1 tsp.
- Whole wheat flour: 3 tbsp.
- Fresh basil or parsley
- 3 tbsp. parmesan cheese, finely grated
- 1 egg mix with 1 tbsp. of water

Instructions

- Slice the eggplant into half-inch-thick slices. Rub salt on pieces and let them rest for 10 to 15 minutes.
- In a bowl, mix the flour with egg + water.
- In a bowl, mix the parmesan cheese, salt, bread crumbs, and Italian seasoning.
- Coat eggplant slices in egg batter, then in bread crumbs mix. Spray with cooking oil.
- Put these slices in an oiled air fryer basket and cook for 8 minutes at 360 F.
- Add one tbsp. of marinara sauce on each piece and cheese. Cook for 1 to 2 more minutes.
- Serve with pasta.

40. Chicken Nuggets

(Ready in about 20 minutes| Serving 4| Difficulty: Medium)

Nutrition per serving: Calories 396|Carbs 17 g| Protein 28 g |Fat 4 g

Ingredients

- 1 and a half cup panko
- 2 chicken breasts, slice into 1"-1.5" pieces
- Parmesan: 1/4 cup
- Sweet paprika: 2 tsp
- Olive oil: 1/3 cup or more

Instructions

- In a bowl, mix parmesan, paprika, and panko.
- Oil spray the air fryer's basket.
- Coat the chicken cubes in olive oil then in panko mix. Coat all the chicken cubes.
- Place them in the air fryer basket in one even layer.
- Cook for 8 minutes at 400 F, until they are cooked and crispy.
- Serve right away.

41. Macaroni & Cheese Balls

(Ready in about 50 minutes| Serving 6-7| Difficulty: Medium)

Nutrition per serving: Calories 213|Carbs 16 g| Protein 4 g |Fat 8 g

Ingredients

- 2 whole eggs
- 1 tsp. of paprika
- 2 tbsp. of milk
- Japanese Panko: 1 cup
- 1 tsp. of salt
- Refrigerated macaroni and cheese: 4 cups
- 2 bacon slices cooked, diced
- Half tsp. of garlic powder

Instructions

- Take 2 tbsp. of macaroni and cheese, make into balls. Set them aside.
- In a mixing bowl, mix milk and egg.
- In another bowl, mix all seasoning and bacon with bread crumbs.
- Coat the mac and cheese balls in egg, then in bread crumbs mix, and place on a baking sheet. Freeze for half an hour.
- Let the air fryer preheat to 360 F.
- Place the coated balls in the basket of the air fryer in one even layer.
- Cook until golden brown or for 8 to 10 minutes.

- Serve right away and enjoy.

42. Greek Turkey Burgers

(Ready in about 25 minutes| Serving 2|Difficulty: Medium)

Nutrition per serving: Calories 351|Carbs 26 g| Protein 28 g |Fat 16 g

Ingredients

- 8 oz. ground turkey breast
- Baby spinach leaves: half cup
- Crushed red pepper: half tsp.
- Olive oil: 1 and a half tbsp.
- Salt: ¼ teaspoon
- Red-wine vinegar: half tsp.
- 2 cloves of minced garlic
- 2 burger buns, toasted
- Red onion: ¼ cup, cut into thin slices
- Fresh oregano, chopped: 2 tsp.
- Feta cheese, crumbled: ¼ cup

Instructions

- Oil spray the air fryer's basket.

- In a bowl, mix ground meat with oil, salt, garlic, oregano, and red pepper. Mix well and shape into two patties.
- Cook at 360 F, for 13-15 minutes in the air fryer, until the internal temperature of patties reaches 155 F.
- In a bowl, onion and spinach with vinegar.
- Put feta on burger buns, add patties and top with vegetable mix and serve.

Chapter 3: Air-Fry Breakfast Recipes

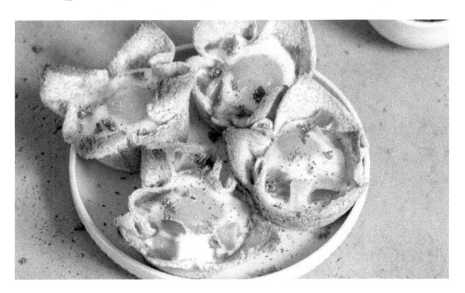

1. French Toast Sticks

(Ready in about 30 minutes| Serving 6-7| Difficulty: Medium)

Nutrition per serving: Calories 170|Carbs 21 g| Protein 6 g |Fat 8 g

Ingredients

- Vanilla extract: 1 tsp.
- 12 slices of Texas toast
- 5 whole eggs
- Cinnamon: 1 tbsp.
- Granulated sugar: 1/4 cup

- Milk: 1 cup
- Melted butter: 4 tbsp.

Instructions

- Cut each bread slice into 3 pieces.
- In a bowl, mix vanilla, milk, butter, and eggs. Whisk well.
- In another bowl mix sugar with cinnamon.
- Coat each stick of bread in the egg mix, then sprinkle with the cinnamon mix.
- Place breadsticks in an oiled basket of air fryer and cook until they get crispy or for 8 minutes at 350 F.
- Serve with syrup.

2. Breakfast Casserole

(Ready in about 35 minutes| Serving 8| Difficulty: Medium)

Nutrition per serving: Calories 280|Carbs 15 g| Protein 12 g |Fat 23 g

Ingredients

- 1 tsp. of Fennel Seed
- 1 lb. of ground sausage
- Half cup of shredded Jack Cheese

- 1 chopped green bell pepper
- Diced white onion: 1/4 cup
- Half tsp. of garlic salt
- 8 eggs, whisked

Instructions

- In a skillet, brown the beef with onions and pepper until vegetables are tender and meat is no longer pink,
- Oil spray the air fryer's basket.
- Take a small dish that is air fryer safe and add sausage mix at the bottom.
- Add cheese on top, and pour whisked eggs on top.
- Sprinkle with garlic salt and fennel seed.
- Place in the air fryer basket, cook at 390 F for 15 minutes.
- Take out the dish and serve.

3. Breakfast Sausage

(Ready in about 20 minutes| Serving 8| Difficulty: Medium)

Nutrition per serving: Calories 173|Carbs 8 g| Protein 13 g |Fat 7 g

Ingredients

- 1 tbsp. of maple syrup
- 1 lb. of ground pork
- 1 tsp. of sea salt
- 1 lb. of ground turkey
- 2 tsp. of fennel seeds
- 2 tsp. of garlic powder
- 1 tsp. of paprika
- 2 tsp. of dry rubbed sage
- 1 tsp. of dried thyme

Instructions

- In a bowl, mix turkey and pork.
- In another bowl, mix the rest of the ingredients.
- Mix the spices with ground meat. Mix well.
- Make 2 to 3 tbsp. into balls and then make into patties.
- Place into the basket of air fryer in one even layer, and cook for ten minutes at 370 F.
- Take out from air fryer and serve with English biscuits.

4. Breakfast Stuffed Peppers

(Ready in about 20 minutes| Serving 2| Difficulty: Medium)

Nutrition per serving: Calories 164|Carbs 4 g| Protein 11 g |Fat 10 g

Ingredients

- olive oil: 1 tsp.
- 1 bell pepper cut into half, remove seeds
- Sriracha flakes: 1 pinch
- 4 whole eggs
- Salt & pepper: 1 pinch of each

Instructions

- Rub the cut side of bell pepper with oil.
- Add 2 eggs in every half of pepper—season with your favorite seasoning.
- Oil spray the air fryer's basket.
- Place peppers in the basket of the air fryer without crowding the basket.
- Cook for 15 minutes at 330 F, or till the eggs reached the desired consistency.

5. Bacon & Egg Breakfast Bombs

(Ready in about 50 minutes| Serving 8| Difficulty: Medium)

Nutrition per serving: Calories 215|Carbs 11 g| Protein 9 g |Fat 9.9 g

Ingredients

- ¼ tsp. of black pepper
- 4 bacon slices, slice into half" pieces
- 1 tbsp. of butter
- 1 egg mixed with 1 tbsp. of water
- 1/4 cup of sharp cheddar cheese, slice into ¾" cubes (10 cubes)
- 2 eggs, whisked
- Buttermilk biscuits, refrigerated (1 can) (5 biscuits)

Instructions

- Cut out a parchment paper of air fryer's basket size and place in the basket and spray the paper with cooking spray.
- In a skillet, cook bacon until it becomes crispy. Take out on a paper towel. Drain the fat.
- Add butter into the skillet, melt the butter.
- Whisk 2 eggs with black pepper.

- Pour eggs into the skillet and cook until still moist. Turn off the heat and add bacon. Let it cool for five minutes.
- Separate 5 biscuits into two layers.
- Add one tbsp. of eggs into each biscuit. Add cheese on top.
- Fold pinch the edges.
- Brush each biscuit bomb with egg wash.
- Place bombs in the basket of air fryer seam side down in one layer.
- Cook for 8 minutes at 325 F; cook for 4 to 6 minutes more if required.

6. Breakfast Potatoes

(Ready in about 40 minutes| Serving 4| Difficulty: Medium)

Nutrition per serving: Calories 232|Carbs 16 g| Protein 9 g |Fat 8 g

Ingredients

- Olive oil: 1 tbsp.
- 1 and a half pounds of potatoes, cut into cubes
- 1 green bell pepper, diced
- Half tsp. of paprika

- 2 minced cloves of garlic
- Half tsp. of salt
- 1/4 of onion, chopped
- Black pepper: 1/4 tsp.

Instructions

- Soak the diced potatoes in the water for half an hour, then take out the potatoes and pat them dry.
- Chop the bell pepper and onion.
- In a bowl, add all ingredients and mix well.
- Place all of it in the air fryer basket and cook for ten minutes at 390 F.
- Shake the air fryer's basket and cook for ten more minutes; shake the air fryer's basket again and cook for five minutes.
- Serve right away.

7. Egg in A Hole

(Ready in about 20 minutes| Serving 1| Difficulty: Easy)

Nutrition per serving: Calories 109|Carbs 7 g| Protein 6 g |Fat 5 g

Ingredients

- 1 slice of bread
- Salt & pepper, to taste

- 1 whole egg

Instructions

- Oil spray the air fryer's basket.
- Make a hole in the center of the bread with a cup cutter.
- Place the bread in an air fryer safe pan and crack an egg in the middle.
- Air fry for 6 minutes at 330 F, turn the bread piece, and cook for 3 to 4 minutes more.
- Serve right away.

8. Baked Eggs Cups

(Ready in about 20 minutes| Serving 1| Difficulty: Easy)

Nutrition per serving: Calories 115|Carbs 1 g| Protein 10 g |Fat 7 g

Ingredients

- 1 whole egg
- Salt & black pepper, to taste
- 1 tbsp. of thawed spinach
- 1 tbsp. of milk
- 1 to 2 tsp. of grated cheese

Instructions

- Spray the ramekin with cooking oil.
- Add egg, spinach, milk, and cheese into the ramekin.
- Sprinkle black pepper and salt. Mix the ingredients but do not break the yolk.
- Cook for 6 to 12 minutes at 330 F; cooking time depends upon the consistency of the egg you want.
- Serve right away and enjoy.

9. Cheesy Chicken Omelet

(Ready in about 25 minutes| Serving 2| Difficulty: Easy)

Nutrition per serving: Calories 115|Carbs 1 g| Protein 10 g |Fat 7 g

Ingredients

- 1/4 tsp. of pepper
- Half cup oven cooked roasted chicken breast, Diced
- 2 tbsp. of cheese, shredded
- 1/4 tsp. of onion powder
- 4 whole eggs
- Half tsp. of salt
- 1/4 tsp. of granulated garlic

Instructions

- Take 2 ramekins and spray them with cooking oil.

- Add 2 eggs to each ramekin.
- Add seasonings (half in one and a half in another) and cheese in each ramekin, whisk well.
- Add in ¼ cup of diced chicken to each ramekin.
- Cook for 14 to 18 minutes at 330 F.
- Serve right away.

10. French Toast Cups with fruits

(Ready in about 40 minutes| Serving 2| Difficulty: Medium)

Nutrition per serving: Calories 406|Carbs 50 g| Protein 14 g |Fat 18 g

Ingredients

- 2 eggs
- 2 pieces of Italian bread, slice into half" cubes
- 1 tbsp. of maple syrup
- ¼ cup of cream cheese, slice into half "cubes
- Half cup of raspberries
- Half cup of whole milk

Syrup

- 1 tbsp. of maple syrup
- Half tsp. of grated lemon zest

- 1/3 cup of water
- 2 cups of raspberries
- 2 tsp. of cornstarch
- Ground cinnamon
- 1 tbsp. of lemon juice

Instructions

- Take 2 custard cups and add half of the bread cubes in these oiled cups.
- Add cream cheese and raspberries.
- Add the rest of the bread on top.
- In a bowl, mix eggs with syrup and milk and pour in custard cups.
- Keep in the fridge for one hour.
- Let the air fryer preheat to 325 F.
- Put custard cups in the air fryer and cook for 12 to 15 minutes until they become puffy and golden brown.
- In a pan, mix water and cornstarch. Add 1 to one and a half cups of raspberries, syrup, lemon zest, and lemon juice.
- Let it boil, turn the heat low and cook for two minutes until thickens.
- Strain it and set it aside.
- Add the rest of the berries into syrup.

- Serve with custard cups and enjoy.

11. Breakfast Burritos

(Ready in about 20 minutes| Serving 6| Difficulty: Medium)

Nutrition per serving: Calories 226|Carbs 12 g| Protein 14 g |Fat 9 g

Ingredients

- Half minced bell pepper
- 6 flour tortillas
- Half cup of shredded cheese
- Half lb. of ground cooked sausage
- 6 eggs, scrambled
- 1/3 cup of bacon bits

Instructions

- In a bowl, mix sausage, cheese, bacon bits, scrambled eggs, and bell pepper. Mix well.
- In a flour tortilla, add a half cup of the mix in the middle.
- Fold the sides and roll tightly.
- Repeat with the rest.
- Place breakfast burritos in the basket of air fryer and spray with cooking oil.

- Cook for 5 minutes at 330 degrees.
- Serve and enjoy.

12. Breakfast Hash

(Ready in about 40 minutes| Serving 4| Difficulty: Medium)

Nutrition per serving: Calories 175|Carbs 23 g| Protein 3 g |Fat 7 g

Ingredients

- 1 tsp. of thyme
- 1 sweet potato, cut into cubes
- 2 tbsp. of olive oil
- 2 russet potatoes, cut into cubes
- 1 yellow onion, cut into cubes
- Half tsp. of pepper
- 2 tsp. of garlic powder
- 1 tsp. of salt

Instructions

- Combine onion and potatoes cubes with garlic powder, olive oil, thyme, pepper, and 2 tbsp. of salt.
- Place this mix into the basket of the air fryer.

- Cook for 20 to 30 minutes at 400 F. Keep checking the mixture and spray with oil if required.
- The hash should be crispy and light brown.

13. Cheese & Veggie Egg Cups

(Ready in about 40 minutes| Serving 4| Difficulty: Medium)

Nutrition per serving: Calories 195|Carbs 7 g| Protein 13 g |Fat 6 g

Ingredients

- 1 tbsp. of minced cilantro
- 1 cup of diced any vegetables
- 4 whole eggs
- 1 cup of shredded cheese
- Salt & black pepper, to taste
- 4 tbsp. of cream

Instructions

- Take four ramekins, and coat them will oil spray.
- In a bowl, mix eggs with half cheese, cilantro, black pepper, salt, cream, and vegetables.
- Pour the mixture in all ramekins equally.
- Place ramekins in the basket of air fryer and cook for 12 minutes at 300 F.

- Add cheese on top and cook for 2 minutes more at 400 F.
- Serve right away.

14. Air Fryer Frittata

(Ready in about 10 minutes| Serving 4| Difficulty: Medium)

Nutrition per serving: Calories 162|Carbs 4 g| Protein 12 g |Fat 10 g

Ingredients

- 1/4 bell pepper chopped
- 3 whole eggs
- 1/4 diced small onion
- 2 tbsp. of shredded cheese
- 2 Cremini mushrooms
- 2 tbsp. of cream
- Salt & pepper, to taste

Instructions

- Mix eggs with salt, cream, and black pepper. Add the vegetables.
- Let the air fryer preheat to 400 F.
- Add the egg mixture to a pan and place it in the air fryer—Cook at 400 F for five minutes.
- Add cheese on top and cook for one more minute.

- Take out the pan, and serve with tomatoes, bread, and avocado.
- Enjoy.

Chapter 4: Air-Fry Poultry Recipes

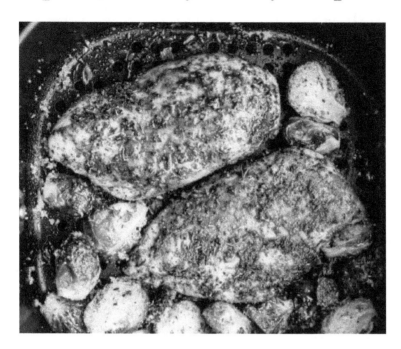

1. Keto Chicken Wings

(Ready in about 20 minutes| Serving 5| Difficulty: Easy)

Nutrition per serving: Calories 220|Carbs 1.2 g| Protein 18 g |Fat 15 g

Ingredients

- 2 tsp. of olive oil
- 3 pounds of chicken wings
- 1 tbsp. of taco seasoning mix

Instructions

- In a resalable bag, add all ingredients. Shake well.
- Let the air fryer preheat to 350 F.
- Put chicken wings in an oiled basket of air fryer and cook for 12 minutes.
- Flip them and cook for six more minutes.
- Serve right away.

2. Southern-Style Chicken

(Ready in about 35 minutes| Serving 6| Difficulty: Medium)

Nutrition per serving (5 ounces): Calories 410|Carbs 13 g|
Protein 36 g |Fat 23 g

Ingredients

- Minced fresh parsley: 1 tbsp.
- 2 cups of crushed Ritz crackers
- Rubbed sage: 1/4 tsp.
- Paprika: 1 tsp.
- Half tsp. Of pepper
- 1 broiler chicken (3-4 pounds), cut up
- Garlic salt: 1 tsp.
- Ground cumin: 1/4 tsp.
- 1 egg, whisked

Instructions

- Let the air fryer preheat to 375 F.
- In a bowl, add whisked egg.
- In another bowl, add crackers and all spices.
- Coat chicken pieces in egg then in cracker mix. Make sure the chicken is coated well spray with cooking oil.
- Put chicken pieces in one even layer in the basket of the air fryer.
- Cook for ten minutes. Flip the chicken and spray with cooking oil; cook for 10 to 20 minutes more until it reaches 165 F and becomes crispy and golden brown.

3. Buttermilk Fried Chicken

(Ready in about 50 minutes| Serving 6| Difficulty: Medium)

Nutrition per serving (5 ounces): Calories 432|Carbs 9 g| Protein 35 g |Fat 23 g

Ingredients

- 1 tbsp. + 1 tsp. of kosher salt
- 1 (3-4 pound) whole chicken
- All-purpose flour: 2 cups
- 1 tsp. of cayenne pepper
- 1 tbsp. of garlic powder
- 1 tsp. of black pepper

- Buttermilk: 2 cups
- 1 tbsp. of ground mustard
- 2 tbsp. of paprika
- 1 tbsp. of onion powder

Instructions

- Cut chicken into ten pieces.
- In a bowl, add all chicken pieces with half tsp. of black pepper, and 1 tsp. of salt.
- Add two cups of buttermilk, mix well, and keep in the fridge for one hour.
- In another bowl, mix half tsp. of pepper, all-purpose flour, 1 tbsp. of salt, ground mustard, and all other spices.
- Let the air fryer preheat to 390 F. Take the chicken out from buttermilk and coat in the flour spice mixture.
- Place chicken pieces in one even layer in the air fryer basket. Flip the chicken halfway through and cook for 18-20 minutes, until internal temperature reaches 165 F.
- Cook the rest of the chicken and serve.

4. Mediterranean Chicken Bowls

(Ready in about 30 minutes| Serving 2-4| Difficulty: Medium)

Nutrition per serving: Calories 475|Carbs 53 g| Protein 43 g |Fat 9 g

Ingredients

- 1 lb. of skinless chicken breasts, boneless, cut into one and a half" pieces
- 2 cups of cherry or grape tomatoes
- Dried oregano: 1 tsp.
- Olive oil: 1 tbsp.
- 1 cup of couscous
- Salt & pepper, to taste
- 1/4 cup of fresh dill
- Ground sumac: 1 tsp.
- 1 chopped onion
- Grated lemon zest: 1 tsp. + 1 Tbsp. of lemon juice
- For serving: feta (crumbled)

Instructions

- In a bowl, coat chicken with oil, half tsp. salt and pepper, sumac, and oregano.
- Add onions and tomatoes, mix well.
- Place in the basket of air fryer and cook at 400 F, for 15-20 minutes, shake the basket a few times until chicken is cooked completely and golden brown.

- In the meantime, mix the couscous with zest and cook as per instructions on the package.
- Fluff it and add in 2 tbsp. of dill and lemon juice.
- Serve couscous with vegetables and chicken. Top with feta and dill, enjoy.

5. Tender Chicken

(Ready in about 8 hours & 20 minutes| Serving 4| Difficulty: Hard)

Nutrition per serving: Calories 275|Carbs 13 g| Protein 13 g |Fat 9 g

Ingredients

- 4 chicken bone-in thighs
- 1 tbsp. smoked paprika
- 1 and a half tbsp. of canola oil
- 1 and a half tsp. of dried rosemary
- 1 and a half tbsp. of whole-grain mustard
- Kosher salt & black pepper, to taste
- 1 lemon, juiced & zested

Instructions

- In a bowl, mix rosemary, mustard, lemon juice, paprika, and zest.

- Coat the chicken in spices. Cover it and keep in the fridge for 4 to 8 hours.

- Let the air fryer preheat to 400 F.

- Take chicken out from marinade.

- Place the chicken in the air fryer, in one even layer. Cook for 18 minutes, and flip halfway through until internal chicken temperature reaches 160 to 165 F.

- Rest the thighs in aluminum for five minutes, then serve and enjoy.

6. Chicken Tikka Skewers with Creamy Avocado Sauce

(Ready in about 2 hours & 20 minutes| Serving 4| Difficulty: Hard)

Nutrition per serving: Calories 232|Carbs 12 g| Protein 11 g |Fat 8.9 g

For Chicken

- 1 lb. of skinless chicken thighs, boneless (slice into bite-size pieces)
- Lemon juice: 1 tbsp.
- Half tsp. of Sea salt
- Half tsp. of Ground cumin

- Avocado mayo: 2 tbsp.
- Freshly grated ginger: 1 tbsp.
- 1 tsp. of Chinese five-spice
- 1/4 tsp. of Coriander
- 1 tsp. of turmeric
- 1 and a half tsp. Smoked paprika
- 2 minced cloves of garlic

Others

- Salt & pepper, to taste
- 1 bell pepper cut julienne style
- 1 onion cut into slices
- Olive oil, as needed

Avocado sauce

- Avocado oil: 2 tbsp.
- Half avocado
- Cilantro leaves: 1/4 cup
- Salt, to taste
- Lime juice: 1 tbsp.
- Water, as needed
- 1 clove of garlic
- Nut milk: 1/4 cup

Instructions

- In a bowl, add chicken and all the other ingredients. Mix well and keep in the fridge for two hours.
- Thread the chicken on skewers, add 2 to 3 pieces of chicken on every skewer.
- Oil spray the air fryer's basket. Put skewers in the basket in one even layer.
- In the air fryer basket, add onion and bell pepper slices in one layer. Pour olive oil over them and season with salt and pepper.
- Select dual cook, and bake the first cycle for five minutes at 350 F.
- Air fry the second cycle for five minutes at 425 F.
- Make sure chicken is cooked, and vegetables are tender.
- In a food processor, add all avocado sauce's ingredients and pulse till it becomes smooth.
- As the food processor is on, add water to make it smooth start with 2 tbsp. of water.
- Add salt to taste.
- Serve the chicken with avocado sauce and with cauliflower rice.

7. Chinese Egg Rolls

(Ready in about 1 hour | Serving 11| Difficulty: Hard)

Nutrition per serving: Calories 215|Carbs 8 g| Protein 11 g |Fat 7 g

Ingredients

- 1 pound of ground chicken or turkey

- Shredded carrots: 1 cup

- Bean sprouts: 1 cup

- Peanut oil: 2 tbsp.

- Soy sauce: 3 tbsp.

- 4 minced cloves of garlic

- Minced ginger: 1 tbsp.

- Thinly sliced green onions: 1/3 cup

- Shredded Napa cabbage: 2 cups

- Hoisin sauce: 1 tbsp.

- Honey: 1 tsp.

- Egg roll wrappers: 25

- Black pepper: 1/4 tsp.

Instructions

- In a skillet, add one tbsp. of peanut oil, heat it. Add Napa cabbage and carrot and cook for two minutes; keep stirring.
- Add bean sprouts and cook for 60 seconds.
- Add honey and one tbsp. of soy sauce. Cook until liquid evaporates or for 1 minute, take out on a plate.
- Add one tbsp. of oil and sauté ginger and garlic for 30 seconds.
- Add ground meat and cook until it becomes brown; keep breaking the meat.
- Add two tbsp. of soy sauce, black pepper, and hoisin sauce.
- Cook for 2-3 minutes until the liquid has been absorbed, take out in a bowl.
- Add green onion and vegetables to the meat bowl and mix well.
- Place egg roll on a clean surface, one corner towards you, and place meat in the bottom third part of an egg roll. Moist the edges with water and seal them roll tightly.
- Let the air fryer preheat to 390 F. place egg rolls on the air fryer basket in one even layer. Cook for 6 minutes, turn them and cook for another five more minutes.
- Serve with dipping sauce.

8. Asian-Glazed Boneless Chicken Thighs

(Ready in about 2 hours & 35 minutes | Serving 4| Difficulty: Hard)

Nutrition per serving: Calories 297|Carbs 5 g| Protein 45 g |Fat 9 g

Ingredients

- 2 and a half tbsp. balsamic vinegar
- 8 skinless, boneless chicken thighs, cleaned and trimmed
- Honey: 1 tbsp.
- 3 minced cloves of garlic
- Fresh grated ginger: 1 tsp.
- Low sodium soy sauce: 1/4 cup
- 1 scallion, thinly sliced for serving
- Sriracha hot sauce: 1 tsp.

Instructions

- In a bowl, mix soy sauce, ginger, honey, sriracha, balsamic, and garlic. Mix it well.
- In a bowl, add chicken with ¼ cup of marinade, coat chicken well, and let it rest for two hours or more.
- Keep the rest of the marinade safe.
- Let the air fryer preheat to 400 F.

- Place chicken in the air fryer basket, cook for 14 minutes and flip and cook until it's completely cooked through.
- Put the remaining marinade in a pot and cook for 1-2 minutes until it becomes thick.
- Pour over chicken thighs and serve with thinly cut scallions.

9. Chicken Parmesan

(Ready in about 35 minutes | Serving 3| Difficulty: Medium)

Nutrition per serving: Calories 462|Carbs 14 g| Protein 23 g |Fat 17 g

Ingredients

- Half tsp. of marinara sauce
- 3 medium chicken breasts
- Half tsp. of onion powder
- 2 eggs, lightly whisked
- 1/4 cup of parmesan cheese
- Half tsp. of Italian seasoning
- 1/4 cup of bread crumbs
- Half tsp. of shredded mozzarella cheese
- Half tsp. of garlic powder

Instructions

- In two different bowls, add whisked eggs in one; in the other, add garlic powder, parmesan, onion, and bread crumbs.
- Coat chicken breast in egg first, then in bread crumbs mix, shake the excess off.
- Pound the breast if needed to make them all the same size.
- Place breaded chicken in an oil sprayed air fryer basket.
- Cook for 15 to 18 minutes at 360 F, or cook till it is cooked completely.
- Place marinara sauce on chicken and top with cheese. Air fry for two more minutes.
- Serve with Italian seasonings on top.

10. Turkey Breast

(Ready in about 50 minutes | Serving 10| Difficulty: Medium)

Nutrition per serving: Calories 462|Carbs 14 g| Protein 23 g |Fat 17 g

Ingredients

- Olive oil: 2 tbsp.

- Ground sage: 1 tsp.
- 3-4-pound of turkey breast, bone-in
- Half tbsp. of poultry seasoning
- Salt & pepper, to taste
- Dried thyme: 1 tsp.

Instructions

- Coat the turkey breast in olive oil and rub the seasoning into the breast.
- Put the seasoned turkey in the air fryer basket, skin side down.
- Cook at 350 F for 25 minutes.
- Flip the breast and cook for half an hour more, until the turkey breast's internal temperature reaches 165 F.
- Let it rest for ten minutes, slice, and serve.

11. Air Fryer Fried Chicken

(Ready in about 35 minutes | Serving 6| Difficulty: Medium)

Nutrition per serving: Calories 321|Carbs 12 g| Protein 22 g |Fat 14 g

Ingredients

For Marinade

- Half cup of buttermilk
- Half of the whole chicken, cut up (thigh, leg, wing, and breast)
- Half cup of hot sauce

For Seasoning

- Garlic powder: 1 tsp.
- All-purpose flour: ¾ cup
- Onion powder: 1 tsp.
- Italian seasoning: 1 tsp.
- Cayenne pepper: Half tsp.
- Seasoning salt: 2 tsp.

Instructions

- Mix the hot sauce and buttermilk, coat the chicken in this mix.
- Keep in the fridge to marinate for 1 to 24 hours.
- In a bowl, mix all the seasoning ingredients and set it aside.
- In the basket of the air fryer, place the parchment paper.
- Take chicken out of buttermilk and coat it in the flour mix.
- Put the breaded chicken in the basket of air fryer in one even layer.

- Cook for 25 minutes at 390 F.
- After 14 minutes, spray the chicken with oil, flip the chicken and cook for 12 minutes more until the chicken's internal temperature reaches 165 F.
- Serve right away.

12. General Tso's Chicken

(Ready in about 26 minutes | Serving 4| Difficulty: Medium)

Nutrition per serving: Calories 265|Carbs 8 g| Protein 23 g |Fat 9 g

Ingredients

For sauce

- Half cup chicken broth
- Sesame oil: 3 tsp.
- Soy sauce: 1 tbsp.
- Ginger: half tsp.
- Half tsp. Sriracha
- Hoisin: 1 tbsp.
- Minced garlic: 1 tsp.
- Cornstarch: 1 tbsp.

For chicken

- Soy sauce: 1 tbsp.
- 2 skinless, boneless chicken breasts, slice into one-inch pieces
- Sesame seeds for serving
- Cornstarch: 1 tbsp.
- 1 scallion, thinly sliced for serving

Instructions

- In a pan, add ginger, garlic, and sesame oil.
- Cook for 60 seconds on low flame.
- Add hoisin, broth, sriracha, and soy sauce, and mix well.
- Add in the cornstarch and keep stirring until it thickens.
- Turn off the heat and set it aside.
- In a bowl, mix cornstarch and soy sauce and mix with chicken.
- Spray the chicken with oil and place in the basket.
- Cook for 16 minutes at 400 F.
- Flip the chicken after half time and spray with oil, and cook.
- Right after, toss with sauce and serve with sesame seeds and scallions on top.

13. Fiesta Chicken Tenders

(Ready in about 25 minutes | Serving 4| Difficulty: Medium)

Nutrition per serving: Calories 676|Carbs 45 g| Protein 23 g |Fat 36 g

Ingredients

- 3/4-pound of skinless, boneless chicken breasts
- 1 pack of taco seasoning
- 1/4 tsp. of pepper
- 1 cup of all-purpose flour
- Salsa, as needed
- Half cup of buttermilk
- 3 cups of crushed corn chips

Instructions

- Let the air fryer preheat to 400 F.
- Pound the chicken with a mallet to half" of thickness.
- Slice into one" strips (wide).
- In a bowl, mix pepper and buttermilk. In another bowl, add the flour, and taco seasoning, and crushed corn chips in a third bowl.
- Coat chicken in flour, then in buttermilk, and finally in corn chips.

- Place chicken in oil sprayed basket, in one even layer.
- Cook for 7 to 8 minutes on both sides until it is completely cooked through.
- Serve with salsa or dipping sauce.

14. Szechuan Crispy Duck

(Ready in about 48 hours & 40 minutes | Serving 5-6| Difficulty: Hard)

Nutrition per serving: Calories 376|Carbs 16 g| Protein 33 g |Fat 21 g

Ingredients

- 4 to 5 lbs. of whole duck (Fresh)

For Marinade

- Salt: 2 tbsp.
- Chinese five-spice powder: 1 tsp.
- Szechuan peppercorns: 2 tbsp.

For Seasonings

- 2 green onions (whole), slice into three" lengths
- dry sherry: 3 tbsp.
- 5 slices (quarter) of fresh ginger, smashed

Starch solution

- Light soy sauce: 1 tbsp.
- Cornstarch: 4 tbsp.
- Water: 3 tbsp.

Instructions

- Roast the peppercorn lightly on medium flame. Turn off the heat and make it into powder in a grinder.
- Mix five spices and salt with ground peppercorns.
- Cut the feet, tail, neck, and wings of duck with a sharp knife.
- Season outside of duck with half of the spice mix and massage them into the duck.
- With the remaining spice mix, rub the insides of the duck.
- Place duck on a cooling rack and place it on a baking sheet, cover the duck with parchment paper, and keep in the fridge for 48 hours.
- After these hours, pour dry sherry inside the duck and put green onion, ginger in the duck.
- Boil water and place a large steamer on top—place duck on a bowl and on a streamer, backside down, and steam for two hours.
- Let it air dry for three hours.

- With a sharp knife, cut the duck in half. In a bowl, add all ingredients of starch solution in a bowl and coat the duck in this mix. Dry for ten minutes.
- Let the air fryer preheat to 400 F.
- Drizzle little oil on duck and put in the air fryer, cut in further half if your air fryer's basket is small.
- Air fry for 10 to 15 minutes. Air-fry the rest of the duck and serve.

15. Lemon Pepper Chicken Thighs

(Ready in about 30 minutes | Serving 6| Difficulty: Medium)

Nutrition per serving: Calories 243|Carbs 6 g| Protein 21 g |Fat 9 g

Ingredients

- Half tsp. Garlic Powder
- 6 skinless, boneless chicken thighs
- ¼ tsp. Black Pepper
- 1 and a half tbsp. lemon juice
- Half tsp. Paprika
- Half tbsp. Lemon Pepper Seasoning
- Half tsp. Italian Seasoning

Instructions

- In a mix all the ingredients, except for chicken. Rub the spice mix all over the chicken.
- Place in the basket of air fryer and cook for 15 minutes at 360 F. flip them after half time and cook until the internal temperature of the meat reaches 165 F.
- Serve right away and enjoy.

16. Roasted Turkey Legs

(Ready in about 45 minutes | Serving 2| Difficulty: Medium)

Nutrition per serving: Calories 251|Carbs 17 g| Protein 29 g |Fat 11 g

Ingredients

- Garlic powder: half tsp.
- 1 and a half tsp smoked paprika
- Brown sugar: 1 tsp.
- 2 turkey legs
- Season salt: 1 tsp.

Instructions

- In a bowl, mix all the spices.
- Dry the turkey legs with paper towels.
- Coat the turkey legs with spice rub and rub under the skin too.

- Oil spray the air fryer's basket.
- Place turkey legs in the basket of air fryer and cook for 20 minutes at 400 F.
- Flip the turkey and cook for 20 minutes more.
- Serve right away.

17. Chicken Souvlaki Gyros

(Ready in about 2 hours & 5 minutes | Serving 4| Difficulty: Hard)

Nutrition per serving: Calories 234|Carbs 16 g| Protein 23 g |Fat 12 g

Ingredients

- 1-pound skinless, boneless chicken breasts
- 1 minced clove of garlic
- 4 pita bread
- Italian seasoning: 1 tbsp.
- Extra-virgin olive oil: 1/4 cup
- Half lemon, cut into slices
- Half cup of chopped tomatoes
- Half tsp. of paprika
- 1/4 tsp. of salt

- 1/4 cup of yogurt sauce (cucumber)

- Shredded lettuce: 1 cup

- 1/4 cup of chopped red onion

Instructions

- In a zip lock bag, add Italian seasoning, salt, olive oil, paprika, lemon, and garlic. Mix well and add chicken and shake it. Keep in the fridge for 2 hours.
- Let the air fryer preheat to 360 F.
- Oil spray the air fryer's basket generously.
- Take chicken out and place it in the basket of the air fryer.
- Cook for ten minutes, flip it and for 8 more minutes, let it cook.
- Let it rest for five minutes, cut into slices.
- Put pita bread on a clean surface, add chicken and other vegetables, and a little yogurt sauce.
- Serve right away.

18. Nashville Hot Chicken

(Ready in about 1 hour & 40 minutes | Serving 6| Difficulty: Medium)

Nutrition per serving: Calories 413|Carbs 20 g| Protein 39 g |Fat 21 g

Ingredients

- 2 pounds of chicken tenderloins
- Slices of Dill pickle
- Dill pickle juice: 2 tbsp.
- 1 tsp. salt
- Buttermilk: Half cup
- Hot pepper sauce: 2 tbsp.
- 1 cup of all-purpose flour
- Pepper: Half tsp.
- Chili powder: 1 tsp.
- Olive oil: half cup
- 1 whole egg
- Cayenne pepper: 2 tbsp.
- Half tsp. Garlic powder
- Dark brown sugar: 2 tbsp.
- Paprika: 1 tsp.

Instructions

- In a bowl, mix one tbsp. of each hot sauce and pickle juice with half tsp. of salt.
- Add in chicken and toss it well. Keep in the fridge for one hour; after one hour, discard the marinade.
- Let the air fryer preheat to 375 F.
- In a bowl, mix flour, pepper, and half tsp. of salt.

- In another bowl, add in 1 tbsp. of pickle juice, egg, 1 tbsp. of hot sauce and buttermilk.
- Coat chicken in flour, then in egg mix, again coat in flour.
- Oil spray the air fryer's basket generously.
- Place chicken in air fryer's basket in one even layer, spray the chicken with oil.
- Cook for 5 to 6 minutes, flip it and spray with oil and cook for 5 to 6 minutes more.
- In a bowl, whisk brown sugar, oil, seasonings, and cayenne pepper.
- Drizzle over chicken and serve chicken on the side of pickles.

19. Crispy Curry Drumsticks

(Ready in about 50 minutes | Serving 4| Difficulty: Medium)

Nutrition per serving (2 ounces): Calories 180|Carbs 2 g| Protein 15 g |Fat 13 g

Ingredients

- Half tsp. of onion salt
- 1 pound of chicken drumsticks
- 3/4 tsp. of salt

- Half tsp. of garlic powder
- Fresh cilantro, Minced
- 2 tbsp. of olive oil
- 2 tsp. of curry powder

Instructions

- In a bowl, add chicken and water to cover the chicken.
- Add half tsp. of salt, let it rest for 15 minutes at the kitchen counter. Drain the water, and with a paper towel, dry the chicken.
- Let the air fryer preheat to 375 F. In a bowl, mix ¼ tsp. of salt, curry powder, oil, garlic powder, and onion salt.
- Add chicken to the spice mix and coat well.
- In the basket of air fryer place chicken in one even layer.
- Cook for 15 to 17 minutes or until the internal temperature of the chicken reaches 170 to 175 F.
- Flip the chicken halfway through to ensure uniform cooking.
- Serve and enjoy.

20. Chicken (Peruvian Style)

(Ready in about 1 day & 80 minutes |Serving 4| Difficulty: Hard)

Nutrition per serving: Calories 523|Carbs 6g| Protein 42 g |Fat 11 g

Ingredients

- Extra virgin olive oil: 3 tbsp.
- 4-5 lb. of chicken cleaned & trimmed
- Lime juice: 2 tbsp.
- 6 cloves of garlic
- Dried oregano: 1 tsp.
- Half tbsp. Kosher salt
- Soy sauce: 2 tbsp.
- Brown sugar: 2 tsp.
- Paprika: 2 tsp.
- Cumin: 1 tbsp.
- Black pepper: 1 tsp.

Instructions

- In a food processor, add all ingredients except for chicken and set it aside.
- Coat the chicken in spice mix and inside of the chicken, under the skin also.

- Let it marinate for 6 to 24 hours.
- Put in the basket of air fryer and cook for half an hour at 360 F.
- Flip the chicken and cook for 20 minutes more, cook until the chicken's internal temperature reaches 165 F.
- Rest the chicken for 15 to 20 minutes. Slice and serve.

21. Korean Chicken Wings

(Ready in about 40 minutes |Serving 4| Difficulty: Medium)

Nutrition per serving: Calories 451|Carbs 44 g| Protein 23 g |Fat 19 g

Ingredients

- 2 lbs. of chicken wings
- half tsp of salt
- Corn starch: ¾ cup
- Onion powder: 1 tsp.
- Garlic powder: 1 tsp.

Korean Sauce

- Minced ginger: 1 tsp.
- Korean gochujang chili paste: 2 tbsp.
- Honey: 3 tbsp.
- Half tsp salt

- Soy sauce: 1 tbsp.
- Brown sugar: 2 tbsp.
- Minced garlic: 1 tsp.

Instructions

- In a bowl, add chicken wings and toss with half tsp. of salt, garlic powder, and onion powder.
- Add corn starch and coat well with tongs.
- Shake excess off and place wings in the basket of the air fryer.
- Cook for half an hour at 390 F, flip and cook for ten minutes more.
- Meanwhile, cook the sauce.
- In a pan, add all sauce's ingredients mix well on medium flame. Let it boil and turn the heat low and simmer for 5 minutes.
- Coat the cooked wings in Korean sauce and serve.

22. Chicken Quesadilla

(Ready in about 15 minutes |Serving 1| Difficulty: Easy)

Nutrition per serving: Calories 106|Carbs 7 g| Protein 7 g |Fat 6 g

Ingredients

- Half cup of chicken breast cooked and cubed

- 2 gluten-free, corn tortillas
- Cheddar cheese, grated: 1/3 cup
- Guacamole: 3 tbsp.

Instructions

- Let the air fryer preheat to 325 F.
- Oil spray the air fryer's basket.
- Place tortilla in the basket, add guacamole, cheese, and chicken on top, and cover with another tortilla.
- Secure with a toothpick.
- Depending upon the crispness, you like to cook for 6 to 10 minutes, flip after half time.
- Slice and serve.

23. Breaded Chicken Breast

(Ready in about 20 minutes |Serving 2| Difficulty: Easy)

Nutrition per serving: Calories 167|Carbs 6 g| Protein 29 g |Fat 3 g

Ingredients

- Ground mustard powder: 2 tsp.
- 1 lb. of chicken breast
- Garlic powder: 2 tsp.
- Salt, to taste

- Onion powder: 2 tsp.
- Olive oil: 2 tsp
- Paprika: 2 tsp.
- Half cup Panko
- Seasoning salt: 2 tsp.

Instructions

- Let the air fryer preheat to 400 F.
- Pound the chicken with a mallet to the desired thickness, and dry with a paper towel.
- Coat the chicken in oil and a pinch of salt.
- In a bowl, add the rest of the ingredients and mix well.
- Sprinkle over the chicken and coat the chicken.
- Spray the chicken with oil and place in an oil sprayed basket of air fryer in one even layer.
- Cook for 8 minutes' flip and cook for 6 to 8 more minutes or until the chicken's internal temperature reaches 165 F.

24. Chicken Chimichangas

(Ready in about 35 minutes |Serving 8| Difficulty: Medium)

Nutrition per serving: Calories 311|Carbs 20 g| Protein 33 g |Fat 7 g

Ingredients

- 8 flour tortillas

- Shredded cooked chicken breast: 4 cups

- 1 can of (16 oz.) red enchilada sauce

- 1 can of (4oz.) green chilies, chopped

- 1 onion, finely diced

- Ground cumin: 1 tsp.

- All-purpose flour: 4 tbsp.

- Garlic powder: ¼ tsp.

Toppings

- Cilantro

- Cheddar Cheese

- Greek Yogurt

Instructions

- Let the air fryer preheat to 400 F.

- Add one tsp of oil to a skillet.

- Add chilies and onion to the skillet and cook for two minutes.

- Add enchilada sauce, flour, garlic powder, salt, and cumin. Keep stirring.

- Add in 2 tbsp. of chicken broth or more if the sauce is too thick.

- Turn off the heat.
- Place tortilla on a clean surface and place a half cup of filling in a tortilla, roll tightly.
- Spray the tortillas with oil and place them in the air fryer in one even layer.
- Cook for four minutes at 400 F, flip and cook until slightly browned or for 2 to 3 more minutes.
- Serve and enjoy.

25. Garlic Herb Chicken Breast

(Ready in about 1 hour & 10 minutes |Serving 6| Difficulty: Medium)

Nutrition per serving: Calories 311|Carbs 20 g| Protein 33 g |Fat 7 g

Ingredients

- 2 lb. of chicken breast, skin on
- Chopped thyme, fresh: 1 tsp.
- Kosher salt & black pepper to taste
- Chopped rosemary, freshly: 1 tsp.
- Melted butter: 4 tbsp.
- 3 minced cloves of garlic

Instructions

- Dry the chicken breast and season with black pepper and salt.
- In a bowl, add all the other ingredients and brush over the chicken breast.
- Put in the air fryer basket and cook for 20 minutes at 375 F, flip it after halftime, cook till the chicken's internal temperature reaches 165 F.
- Serve right away and enjoy.

26. Almond Chicken

(Ready in about 30 minutes |Serving 2| Difficulty: Medium)

Nutrition per serving: Calories 353|Carbs 6 g| Protein 41 g |Fat 18 g

Ingredients

- 2 skinless, boneless chicken breast, cut into halves
- Buttermilk: 1/4 cup
- 1 whole egg
- Slivered almonds, finely diced: 1 cup
- Garlic salt: 1 tsp.
- Black pepper: half tsp.

Instructions

- Let the air fryer preheat to 350 F.

- In a bowl, add buttermilk, pepper, garlic salt, and egg.
- In another bowl, add almonds.
- Coat chicken in egg mix then in almonds, pat to coat well.
- Put the chicken in the oil sprayed basket of the air fryer and spray the chicken with oil also.
- Cook for 15 to 18 minutes, until internal temperature, reaches 165 F.
- Serve with any sauce.

27. Fajita-Stuffed Chicken

(Ready in about 35 minutes |Serving 4| Difficulty: Medium)

Nutrition per serving: Calories 347|Carbs 5 g| Protein 42 g |Fat 17 g

Ingredients

- 4 skinless, boneless chicken breast, cut in half
- Ground cumin: 1 tsp.
- 1 onion, cut into thin slices
- Ground cumin: 1 tsp.
- Olive oil: 1 tbsp.
- Half green pepper, cut into thin slices
- Half cup of cheddar cheese, 4 slices
- Garlic powder: 1/4 tsp.

- Chili powder: 1 tbsp.
- Half tsp. of salt

Instructions

- Let the air fryer preheat to 375 F.
- Make a pocket in the thick part of the chicken breast. Fill it with green pepper and onion.
- In a bowl, mix seasonings and olive oil, coat the chicken in this mix.
- Oil spray the air fryer's basket and place chicken inside, and cook for six minutes.
- Add slices of cheese on top and cook for 6 to 8 more minutes, until the internal temperature of the chicken reaches 165 F.
- Serve and enjoy.

28. Everything Bagel Chicken Strips

(Ready in about 25 minutes |Serving 4| Difficulty: Medium)

Nutrition per serving: Calories 269|Carbs 8 g| Protein 31 g |Fat 13 g

Ingredients

- 1 pound of chicken tenderloins
- Everything bagel, 1 day-old shredded in large pieces
- half cup of Parmesan cheese, grated

- 1/4 tsp. red pepper flakes, crushed
- Half tsp. salt
- Cubed butter: 1/4 cup
- Half cup of panko bread crumbs

Instructions

- Let the air fryer preheat to 400 F. In a food processor, add bagel until it becomes crumby.
- In a bowl, add a half cup of bagel crumbs and add pepper flakes, cheese, and panko.
- Melt the butter. Season chicken with salt, and dip in melted butter.
- Coat in crumbs mix.
- Oil spray the air fryer's basket and place breaded chicken in the basket of the air fryer.
- Cook for seven minutes, then flip the chicken and cook until it becomes golden brown, for 7 to 8 minutes.
- Serve right away.

29. Sweet Chili Chicken Wings

(Ready in about 30 minutes |Serving 4| Difficulty: Medium)

Nutrition per serving: Calories 324|Carbs 12 g| Protein 24 g |Fat 4 g

Ingredient

- Chicken Wings: 12
- Paprika: ¼ tsp.
- Baking powder: Half tbsp.
- Sea salt: half tsp.
- Onion powder: ¼ tsp.
- Black pepper: 1 tsp.
- Garlic powder: 1 tsp.

Sweet Thai Chili Sauce

- Hoisin Sauce: 1 and a half tbsp.
- Soy Sauce: 1 tbsp.
- 3 and a half tbsp. sweet chili sauce
- Lime Juice: half tbsp.
- Rice Wine Vinegar: half tbsp.
- Sesame Oil: half tbsp.
- Sea Salt: ¼ tsp
- Brown Sugar: 1 tbsp.
- 2 minced cloves of garlic
- Water: ¼ Cup
- Ground ginger: half tsp.

Instructions

- In a reseal able bag, add all spices, baking powder with chicken wings.
- Shake the bag and mix well.
- Oil spray the air fryer's basket and place chicken inside in a single layer.
- Cook for 20 minutes at 400 F; after ten minutes, flip the wings.
- Meanwhile, make the sweet chili sauce.
- In a pan, add all the ingredients of the sauce and heat on medium flame.
- Let it boil and turn the heat low; let it simmer until it thickens.
- Coat the wings in sauce and serve.

30. Sesame Chicken

(Ready in about 30 minutes |Serving 6| Difficulty: Medium)

Nutrition per serving: Calories 335|Carbs 28 g| Protein 30 g |Fat 9 g

Ingredients

- Half cup of cornstarch
- 6 skinless boneless, chicken thighs

Sauce

- Cornstarch: 1 tbsp.
- Soy Sauce: 1/4 Cup
- 1 minced clove of garlic
- Orange Juice: 2 tbsp.
- Hoisin Sauce: 5 tsp.
- Brown Sugar: 2 tbsp.
- Ground Ginger: Half tsp.
- Sesame Seeds: 2 tsp.
- Cold Water: 1 tbsp.

Instructions

- Slice the chicken into cubes, add in a bowl add coat in cornstarch.
- Let the air fryer preheat to 390 F.
- Oil spray the chicken and the basket of the air fryer. Cook for 24 minutes, flip the pieces halfway through and spray with oil.
- In a pan, add all sauce ingredients, except for cornstarch, sesame seeds, and water on medium flame.
- Whisk it well. Let it boil and add in the rest of the ingredients. Add seeds in the last.
- Turn off the heat and let it rest for five minutes.
- Coat the chicken with sauce and serve with rice.

31. Apricot Glazed Chicken Drumsticks

(Ready in about 37 minutes |Serving 2| Difficulty: Medium)

Nutrition per serving: Calories 278|Carbs 11 g| Protein 21 g |Fat 9 g

Ingredients

Spicy Apricot Glaze

- Soy sauce: half tsp.
- Half cup of apricot preserves
- Chili powder: 1/4 tsp.
- Dijon mustard: 2 tsp.

For Chicken

- Seasoned salt: half tsp.
- 4-6 chicken drumsticks
- Pepper: Half tsp.
- Salt: 1 tsp.

Instructions

- In a pan, add all ingredients of the sauce and whisk well on low flame until it becomes thick, for 5-10 minutes. Turn off the heat and set it aside.
- Oil spray the air fryer's basket and chicken.
- In a bowl, mix seasoned salt, black pepper, and salt.

- Sprinkle the spice mix on chicken and place in the basket of the air fryer.
- Cook for ten minutes at 370 F, flip the chicken and spray with oil.
- Cook for ten more minutes.
- Take chicken out and brush with sauce, cook for two more minutes and serve.

32. Honey Garlic Chicken

(Ready in about 37 minutes |Serving 4| Difficulty: Medium)

Nutrition per serving: Calories 629|Carbs 76 g| Protein 40 g |Fat 13 g

Ingredients

- 6 skinless, boneless chicken thighs
- Soy Sauce: half cup
- Potato starch, as needed
- Cornstarch: 1 tbsp.
- Ketchup: 2 tbsp.
- Honey: half cup
- Sliced green onions
- Cooked green beans
- 1 minced clove of garlic
- Brown Sugar: 2 tbsp.

- Ground Ginger: half tsp.
- Cooked Rice

Instructions

- Slice the chicken into cubes and coat with potato starch.
- Cook in the air fryer for 12 minutes, at 390 F, flip and cook for 12 minutes more.
- In a pan, add ketchup, honey, brown sugar, soy sauce, ginger, and garlic.
- Let it boil on low heat. Add in cornstarch until it becomes thick.
- Add cooked chicken in the sauce, reheat if required.
- Serve with green beans, rice, and top with green onion.

33. Mongolian Chicken

(Ready in about 45 minutes |Serving 4| Difficulty: Medium)

Nutrition per serving: Calories 445|Carbs 56 g| Protein 32 g |Fat 11 g

Ingredients

- Vegetable Oil: 2 tsp.
- 1 pound of skinless, boneless chicken thighs
- Cornstarch: 1/4 Cup
- Brown Sugar Packed: 3/4 Cup

- Minced garlic: 1 tbsp.
- Soy Sauce: half cup
- Ginger: half tsp.
- Water: half cup

Instructions

- Cut chicken into cubes, and toss with cornstarch.
- Place foil in the air fryer basket and spray with oil.
- Place chicken in the foil and spray with oil.
- Cook at 390 F for 12 minutes.
- Toss chicken and spray with oil.
- Cook for 12 more minutes.
- Meanwhile, in a pot, add soy sauce, ginger, sugar, oil, garlic, and water. Mix well.
- Let it boil on low flame. Add in cooked chicken.
- Let it rest for 5 to 10 minutes with the heat turned off.
- Serve the chicken with sautéed vegetables and rice.

34. Chicken Teriyaki Bowls

(Ready in about 50 minutes |Serving 6| Difficulty: Medium)

Nutrition per serving: Calories 404|Carbs 47 g| Protein 35 g |Fat 9 g

Ingredients

- Rice wine vinegar: 2 tbsp.
- 6 skinless, boneless chicken thighs
- Water: 1/4 Cup
- Soy Sauce: half cup
- Granulated sugar: 1/4 Cup
- Cornstarch: 1/4 Cup + half tbsp.
- 1 minced clove of garlic
- Brown sugar: 2 tbsp.
- Cooked white rice: 3 Cups
- Ground ginger: 1 tsp.
- 2 green onions, chopped
- Cooked green beans: 2 Cups

Instructions

- Cut chicken into cubes and toss with cornstarch.
- Cook in the air fryer for 10 to 15 minutes at 390 F.
- In a pan, add brown sugar, ginger, soy sauce, regular sugar, water, garlic, and rice wine vinegar. Mix it well.
- Let it boil on low flame and add in half tbsp. of cornstarch, let it get thick to your desired preference.
- Turn off the heat and let it cool for five minutes.
- Make sure the chicken's internal temperature reaches 165 F.

- Coat the chicken with sauce and serve with white rice, beans and top with green onion.

35. Peach-Bourbon Wings

(Ready in about 50 minutes |Serving 12| Difficulty: Medium)

Nutrition per serving: Calories 79|Carbs 7 g| Protein 5 g |Fat 3 g

Ingredients

- 2 pounds of chicken wings
- Bourbon: 2 tbsp.
- Peach preserves: half cup
- 1 minced clove of garlic
- Water: 1 and a half tsp.
- Salt: 1/4 tsp.
- White vinegar: 2 tbsp.
- Brown sugar: 1 tbsp.
- Cornstarch: 1 tsp.

Instructions

- Let the air fryer preheat to 400 F.
- In a food processor, add garlic, peach preserves, salt, and brown sugar. Pulse until it gets blended.

- Pour in a pan, add bourbon and vinegar on medium flame. Let it boil, turn the heat low and let it simmer for 4 to 6 minutes until it becomes thick.
- In a bowl, add water and cornstarch until smooth; add in the sauce. Let it boil, keep mixing for 1 to 2 minutes.
- Clean the wing tips and discard them.
- Oil spray the air fryer's basket and place wings inside air fryer basket and cook for six minutes, flip and brush with sauce.
- Cook for 6 to 8 minutes until browned.
- Serve wings with sauce.

36. Popcorn Chicken

(Ready in about 50 minutes |Serving 12| Difficulty: Medium)

Nutrition per serving: Calories 79|Carbs 7 g| Protein 5 g |Fat 3 g

Ingredients

Marinade

- Almond milk: 2 cups
- 2 lbs. of chicken tenders, sliced into small pieces
- Half tsp. of ground paprika
- Salt: 1 tsp.

- Half tsp. of black pepper

Dry Ingredients

- Paprika: 2 tsp.
- Flour: 3 cups
- Black pepper: 2 tsp.
- Salt: 3 tsp.

Instructions

- In a reseal able bag, add all the ingredients of marinade and chicken. Seal the bag and shake it well.
- Keep in the fridge for 2-6 hours.
- In a bowl, add all dry ingredients. Mix well.
- Take the chicken and marinade out in a bowl.
- Coat chicken in the spice mix. Lightly coat in marinade and coat in the spice mix.
- Oil spray the air fryer's basket and place chicken in one even layer in the basket.
- Spray the chicken with oil and cook for 10 minutes at 370 F.
- Serve with any sauce and rice.

Chapter 5: Air-Fry Beef & Pork Recipes

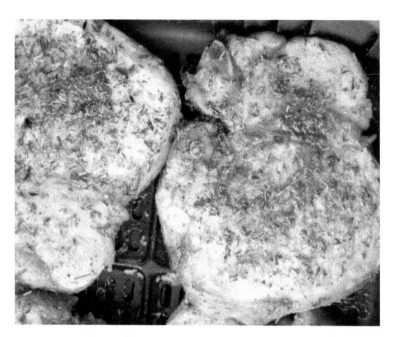

1. Air-Fried Meatloaf

(Ready in about 1 day | Serving 4| Difficulty: Medium)

Nutrition per serving (3 balls): Calories 585|Carbs 30 g| Protein 29 g |Fat 38 g

Ingredient

- Half-pound of ground veal
- 1 egg
- Half pound of ground pork

- Fresh cilantro, chopped: ¼ cup
- 2 spring onions, chopped
- Chipotle chili sauce: 2 tsp.
- Bread crumbs: ¼ cup
- Black pepper: half tsp.
- Sriracha salt: half tsp.
- Molasses: 1 tsp.
- Ketchup: half cup
- Olive oil: 1 tsp.

Instructions

- Let the air fryer preheat to 400 F.
- In a baking dish, mix veal and pork that can be placed in the air fryer.
- Add in black pepper, egg, Sriracha salt (half tsp.), crumbs, cilantro, spring onions.
- With clean hands, mix it well, and make it into a loaf.
- In a bowl, mix olive oil, ketchup, molasses, and chili sauce; mix well.
- Air fry the meatloaf for 25 minutes.
- After 25 minutes, take the meatloaf out and pour the ketchup mix.
- Air fry for seven more minutes, till the internal temperature reaches 160 F.

- Let the loaf rest in the air fryer after Turing it off for five minutes.
- Rest five more minutes, then serve.

2. Ground Beef Wellington

(Ready in about 50 minutes | Serving 4| Difficulty: Medium)

Nutrition per serving (3 balls): Calories 585|Carbs 30 g| Protein 29 g |Fat 38 g

Ingredients

- Half pound of ground beef
- Butter: 1 tbsp.
- All-purpose flour: 2 tbsp.
- Chopped mushrooms: half cup
- Half & half cream: half cup
- 1 egg yolk
- Pepper: 1/4 tsp.
- 1 tube of crescent rolls, refrigerated
- Chopped onion: 2 tbsp.
- Dried parsley: 1 tsp.
- Salt: 1/4 tsp.
- 1 egg, whisked

Instructions

- Let the air fryer preheat to 300 F.
- In a pan, add butter and sauté mushrooms for 5 to 6 minutes, until tender.
- Add in pepper (1/8 tsp.) and flour, mix it well.
- Add cream. Let it boil, mix for two minutes until it thickens.
- Turn off the heat and set it aside.
- In a mixing bowl, mix onion, mushroom mix (2 tbsp.), yolk, rest of the pepper and salt.
- Add to beef mixture and mix it well.
- Make into two loaves.
- Roll the dough and divide into two rectangles. Put loaves in these triangles and wrap them well, seal the edges. Brush with whisked egg.
- Put wellington in the oil sprayed basket of air fryer and cook for 18 to 22 minutes, until internal temperature reaches 160 F.
- Add Parsley in the mushroom sauce and serve with beef wellington.

3. Papas Rellenas

(Ready in about 75 minutes | Serving 6| Difficulty: Hard)

Nutrition per serving (3 balls): Calories 625|Carbs 40 g| Protein 13 g |Fat 46 g

Ingredients

- 2 and a half pounds of peeled potatoes slice into wedges
- 1 onion, chopped
- 1 pound of lean ground beef
- Tomato sauce: half cup
- 1 green pepper, chopped
- Green olives with pimientos sliced: half cup
- 1 and 1/4 tsp. of salt
- Garlic powder: 1 tsp.
- 1 and 1/4 tsp. of pepper
- Bread crumbs, seasoned: 1 cup
- Paprika: half tsp.
- 2 eggs, whisked
- Raisins: half cup

Instructions

- In a large pan, add potatoes and enough water to cover them. Let them boil, turn the heat low cook for 15 to 20 minutes, till tender
- In a skillet, cook onion, beef, and green pepper on medium flame until meat is cooked.
- Add in raisins, salt (1/4 tsp.), paprika, tomato sauce, black pepper (1/4 tsp.), and olives.

- Mash the drained potatoes with salt, black pepper (1 tsp. of each), and garlic.
- Take 2 tbsp. of potato mix and shape into a patty, fill it with one tbsp. of filling.
- Wrap the potato around the filling and make a ball. Keep making potato balls like this.
- In different bowls, add bread crumbs and eggs.
- Coat balls in egg then in bread crumbs.
- Let the air fryer preheat to 400 F.
- Air fry the balls for 14 to 16 minutes until golden brown.
- Serve right away.

4. Taco Twists

(Ready in about 35 minutes | Serving 4|Difficulty: Medium)

Nutrition per serving: Calories 371|Carbs 30 g| Protein 16 g |Fat 21 g

Ingredients

- 1 tube of crescent rolls, refrigerated
- 1/3 pound of ground beef
- Cheddar cheese, shredded: 2/3 cup
- 1 diced onion
- Diced green chilies: 3 tbsp.

- Garlic powder: 1/4 tsp.
- Ground cumin: 1/8 tsp.
- Salsa: 1/3 cup
- Hot pepper sauce: 1/4 tsp.
- Salt: 1/8 tsp.

Instructions

- Let the air fryer preheat to 300 F.
- In a skillet, cook onions and beef on medium flame until meat is fully cooked.
- Add in cumin, cheese, hot pepper sauce, salsa, salt, chilies, and garlic powder.
- Roll the dough and divide into four rectangles; put half a cup of meat mix in every rectangle.
- Make four corners join with each other and twist it.
- Place in an oil sprayed basket of air fryer and cook for 18 to 22 minutes, in one even layer.
- Serve right away.

5. Steak Fajitas

(Ready in about 30 minutes | Serving 6|Difficulty: Medium)

Nutrition per serving: Calories 309|Carbs 29 g| Protein 27 g |Fat 9 g

Ingredients

- 1 beef flank steak
- 6 tortillas, whole wheat
- 2 tomatoes, chopped without seeds
- 1 jalapeno, chopped without seeded
- Chopped red onion: half cup
- Chopped fresh cilantro: 3 tbsp.
- Ground cumin: 2 tsp.
- Lime juice: 1/4 cup
- Salt: 3/4 tsp.
- 1 onion, cut into slices

Instructions

- In a bowl, add jalapenos, chopped red onion, tomatoes, cilantro, lime juice with salt (1/4 tsp.), cumin (1 tsp.), mix well, and set it aside.
- Let the air fryer preheat to 400 F.
- Season steak with the rest of the salt and cumin.
- Put on an oil sprayed basket of air fryer and cook for 6 to 8 minutes on each side until internal temperature reaches 135- 145 F. keep checking for the desired doneness.
- Take out and let it rest for five minutes.
- Air fryer the sliced onion for 2 to 3 minutes.

- Cut the steak into strips or shred the steak.
- Place tortilla on a flat surface and top with salsa, onion, and steak strips.
- Serve right away

6. Herb & Cheese-Stuffed Burgers

(Ready in about 35 minutes | Serving 4|Difficulty: Medium)

Nutrition per serving: Calories 369|Carbs 29 g| Protein 29 g |Fat 14 g

Ingredients

- 1 pound of lean ground beef
- 2 green onions, cut into thin slices
- Dijon mustard: 4 tsp.
- Chopped fresh parsley: 2 tbsp.
- Ketchup: 2 tbsp.
- Dried rosemary: half tsp.
- 4 buns, cut in half
- Dry bread crumbs: 3 tbsp.
- Dried sage leaves: 1/4 tsp.
- 2 oz. of sliced cheddar cheese
- salt: half tsp.

Instructions

- Let the air fryer preheat to 375 F.
- In a bowl, mix mustard (2 tsp.), green onions, and parsley.
- In another bowl, mix mustard (2 tsp.), ketchup, all crumbs, and seasonings. Mix and add beef to this bowl; mix it well but do not overmix.
- Make into eight patties. Put green onion mix and cheese slices on 4 patties.
- Place one patty on top of the filling, seal the edges.
- Cook in oil sprayed basket of air fryer for 8 minutes on one side in one even layer, carefully flip and cook for 6 to 8 minutes more until internal temperature reaches 160 F.
- Place on buns and serve.

7. Juicy Pork Chops

(Ready in about 25 minutes | Serving 4|Difficulty: Medium)

Nutrition per serving: Calories 569|Carbs 17 g| Protein 32 g |Fat 40 g

Ingredients

- Dijon mustard: 1 tbsp.
- 4 center cut, boneless pork chops
- 1 egg

- Onion powder: half tsp.
- Panko breadcrumbs: half cup
- Garlic powder: half tsp.
- Dry breadcrumbs: 1/4 cup
- Kosher salt: 1 tsp.
- Parmesan cheese, grated: 1/4 cup

Instructions

- Let the air fryer preheat to 400 F.
- Sprinkle salt over pork chops and rub lightly.
- In a bowl, mix mustard with egg.
- In a zip lock bag, add garlic powder, all breadcrumbs, onion powder, and Parmesan.
- Shake the bag well.
- Coat pork chops in the egg mix, then in breadcrumbs. Shake the bag to coat evenly.
- Oil spray the air fryer's basket and put 2 chops inside in one layer.
- Cook for six minutes, flip them, and the internal temperature should reach 145 F, and cook for six more minutes.
- Cook the rest and serve.

8. Mini Calzones

(Ready in about 25 minutes | Serving 12|Difficulty: Medium)

Nutrition per serving: Calories 185|Carbs 16.4 g| Protein 8.4 g |Fat 9.3 g

Ingredients

- Pizza sauce: 1 cup
- All-purpose flour, as needed
- Chopped pepperoni: ¾ cup
- 1 pound of pizza dough
- Mozzarella cheese, shredded: 1 cup

Instructions

- Roll the pizza dough on a floured surface to make it ¼" thick. Cut out 8-10 circles of dough (~3" each). You should get 16 pieces.
- On a baking sheet place parchment paper and place circles on it.
- Add 2 tsp. of sauce on each round, 1 tsp. of pepperoni and 1 tsp. of cheese.
- Fold the one half over the filling and seal the edges with a fork.
- Let the air fryer preheat to 375 F.

- Place calzones in the basket of air fryer in one layer and cook for 8 minutes, till they turn golden brown.
- Serve right away.

9. Gingery Pork Meatballs

(Ready in about 45 minutes | Serving 4|Difficulty: Medium)

Nutrition per serving: Calories 620|Carbs 59 g| Protein 26 g |Fat 31.5 g

Ingredients

Noodles

- Half cucumber, slice into matchsticks
- 6 oz. of rice noodles
- 1 carrot, slice into matchsticks
- Sesame dressing: half cup
- 1 scallion, cut into thin slices
- Chopped cilantro: 1/4 cup

Meatballs

- 1 lb. of ground pork
- Grated lime zest: 2 tsp.
- 1 egg
- 1 and a half tbsp. of honey
- Fish sauce: 1 tsp.
- Lime juice: 2 tbsp.

- Grated ginger: 1 tbsp.
- Chopped cilantro: 1/4 cup
- Salt, to taste
- 1 jalapeño, chopped without seeds
- 1 minced clove of garlic
- Panko: half cup
- 2 scallions, chopped

Instructions

- Cook noodles as per package directions. Wash with cold water and mix with the rest of the ingredients. Set it aside.
- In a mixing bowl, add lime juice, salt (half tsp.), fish sauce, egg, honey, zest, and panko. Mix well and let it rest for 60 seconds.
- Add in jalapeño, garlic, ginger, and scallions. Add cilantro and pork mix well.
- Make into 1 tbsp. of meatballs and place in the oil sprayed basket of the air fryer.
- Cook at 400 F for 8 to 12 minutes.
- Serve the meatballs with noodles.

10. Bacon-Roasted Potatoes

(Ready in about 30 minutes | Serving 4|Difficulty: Medium)

Nutrition per serving: Calories 275 |Carbs 35 g| Protein 7 g |Fat 3 g

Ingredients

- 4 sprigs of thyme
- 1 and a half lb. of small potatoes, cut into half
- Salt and pepper, to taste
- Balsamic vinegar: 1 tbsp.
- 3 slices of bacon
- Olive oil: 1 tbsp.
- Whole-grain mustard: 2 tsp.
- 3 shallots, slice into ¼" wedges

Instructions

- In a bowl, add half cut potatoes, black pepper (1/4 tsp.), thyme, and salt (half tsp.)
- Toss well and place in the air fryer and put bacon on top.
- Cook for 6-12 minutes at 400 F, take the bacon out and crumble it.
- Shake the basket and cook for eight more minutes.
- Place shallots in the air fryer and shake the basket, cook for 8 to 12 minutes more.

- In a bowl, add thyme leaves, vinegar, and mustard. Mix and add air fried vegetables and bacon to it. Toss well and serve.

11. Boneless Pork Chop

(Ready in about 20 minutes | Serving 2|Difficulty: Easy)

Nutrition per serving: Calories 258 |Carbs 19 g| Protein 19 g |Fat 11 g

Ingredients

- 2 pork chops (boneless and 1.25-inch thick)
- Pork rub: 2 tsp.
- Salt & black pepper, to taste

Instructions

- Let the air fryer preheat to 400 F.
- Season the pork with pork rub and a little salt and black pepper.
- Put chops in the air fryer and cook for six minutes.
- Turn the chops and cook for 5 to 8 minutes until the chops' internal temperature reaches 135 to 145 F.
- Let the chops rest before serving.

12. Panko Crusted Pork Chops

(Ready in about 22 minutes | Serving 4|Difficulty: Medium)

Nutrition per serving: Calories 258 |Carbs 19 g| Protein 19 g |Fat 11 g

Ingredients

- 2-4 boneless, center-cut pork chops
- Chili powder: half tsp.
- Salt: ¼ tsp.
- 1 whisked egg
- Parmesan cheese: 1 tbsp.
- Onion powder: half tsp.
- Paprika: 1 and a half tsp.
- Panko: 1 cup
- Granulated garlic: 1 and a half tsp.
- Pepper: ¼ tsp.

Instructions

- Let the air fryer preheat to 400 F.
- Season chops with salt.
- In a bowl, add whisked egg.
- In another bowl, mix black pepper, panko, cheese, chili powder, paprika, onion powder, and garlic.
- Coat the chops in egg then in bread crumbs.
- Oil spray the air fryer's basket and place breaded chops inside and spray them with oil.

- Cook for 12 minutes at 400 F.
- Turn the chops after halfway through, oil spray them again.
- Serve right away.

13. Cheeseburger

(Ready in about 40 minutes | Serving 8|Difficulty: Medium)

Nutrition per serving: Calories 258 |Carbs 19 g| Protein 19 g |Fat 11 g

Ingredients

- All-purpose flour: 3/4 cup
- 1 and a half cups of bread crumbs
- 1 pound of lean ground beef
- Mustard: 2 tbsp.
- Ketchup: 1/3 cup
- 1 onion (large)
- 4 oz. Of cheddar cheese, diced
- Salt: half tsp.
- 2 eggs, lightly whisked
- Garlic powder: 2 tsp.

Instructions

- Let the air fryer preheat to 335 F.
- In a bowl, mix ketchup, salt, beef, and mustard. Mix it well but do not over mix.
- Slice onion into rounds, and fill with the beef mix (only 8 rings).
- Add cheese cubes and beef on top.
- In a bowl, mix garlic powder and flour.
- In another bowl, mix eggs. In the third bowl, add bread crumbs.
- Coat filled onion rings in flour, then in egg mixture, and lastly in crumbs.
- Oil spray the air fryer's basket and place onion rings in the air fryer basket and spray with oil.
- Cook for 12 to 15 minutes or the internal temperature of the meat reaches 160 F.
- Serve right away and enjoy.

14. Loaded Pork Burritos

(Ready in about 40 minutes | Serving 6|Difficulty: Medium)

Nutrition per serving: Calories 910 |Carbs 82 g| Protein 50 g |Fat 42 g

Ingredients

- Olive oil: 1 tbsp.
- Salt: 2 tsp.
- Concentrate limeade: 3/4 cup
- 1 and a half tsp. Of pepper
- Chopped plum tomatoes: 1 cup (without seeds)
- 1 diced green pepper
- 1 and a half pounds of pork loin, (boneless) thinly cut strips
- 1 diced onion
- 1 can of (15 oz.) Black beans, drained & rinsed
- 1 jalapeno chopped without seeds
- Chopped fresh cilantro: 1/4 cup + 1/3 cup
- 6 flour tortillas (12")
- Jack cheese, shredded: 3 cups
- Lime juice: 1 tbsp.
- Garlic powder: 1/4 tsp.
- Uncooked rice, long grain: 1 cup
- 1 and a half cups of sour cream

Instructions

- In a bowl, mix salt (1 tsp.), concentrate limeade, and half tsp. of pepper, mix well, and add pork. Coat well and keep in the fridge for 20 minutes.

- In a bowl, add green pepper, jalapeno, black pepper, cilantro (1/4 cup), tomatoes, black pepper, onion, garlic powder, salt, and lime juice. Mix well and set it aside.
- Cook rice as per package directions. Add in cilantro and mix.
- Let the air fryer preheat to 350 F.
- Oil spray the air fryer's basket and place pork inside in one even layer and spray with oil. Cook for 8 to 10 minutes, flipping halfway through.
- Lay warmed tortilla on a clean surface, place cheese (1/3 cup), not in the middle, prepared salsa (1/4 cup), sour cream (1/4 cup), beans (1/4 cup), half cup of rice, and a half cup of pork on top.
- Roll tightly and serve.

15. Pork Schnitzel

(Ready in about 30 minutes | Serving 4|Difficulty: Medium)

Nutrition per serving: Calories 309 |Carbs 17 g| Protein 30 g |Fat 13 g

Ingredients

- Pork sirloin cutlets: 4 (4 oz. Each)

- All-purpose flour: 1/4 cup
- Black pepper: 1/4 tsp.
- 1 egg
- Paprika: 1 tsp.
- Seasoned salt: 1 tsp.
- Milk: 2 tbsp.
- Bread crumbs, dry: 3/4 cup

Dill sauce

- Chicken broth: 3/4 cup
- All-purpose flour: 1 tbsp.
- Dill weed: 1/4 tsp.
- Sour cream: half cup

Instructions

- Let the air fryer preheat to 375 F.
- In a bowl, mix black pepper, flour, and seasoned salt.
- In a separate bowl, mix milk with egg.
- In another bowl, mix paprika and bread crumbs.
- Pound the cutlets with a mallet to make them ¼" thick.
- Coat the pork in flour, then in the egg mix, and lastly in bread crumbs. Coat them well.

- Oil spray the air fryer's basket and place cutlets inside in one even layer and spray with oil, cook for 4 to 5 minutes, flip and cook for 5 more minutes
- In a pan, mix broth and flour until well combined. Let it boil and keep mixing, cook for two minutes.
- Turn heat to low and add in dill and sour cream, do not let it boil.
- Serve the cutlets with dill sauce.

16. Beef Short Ribs

(Ready in about 1 hour & 20 minutes | Serving 4|Difficulty: Hard)

Nutrition per serving: Calories 245 |Carbs 1 g| Protein 31 g |Fat 3 g

Ingredients

- 1 pound of beef short ribs
- Soy sauce: 2 tbsp.
- 2 crushed cloves of garlic
- Brown sugar: 2 tbsp.
- Sesame oil: 1 tbsp.
- Ground ginger: 1 tsp.

Instructions

- In a bowl, mix ginger, soy sauce, brown sugar, and sesame oil.
- In a zip lock bag, add the ribs, ginger mix, and crushed cloves.
- Toss it well and keep it in the fridge for 1-24 hours.
- Let the air fryer preheat to 300 F.
- Oil spray the air fryer's basket, place ribs inside in one layer, leaving room in between.
- Cook for a total of 20 minutes, flip after halfway through.
- Take ribs out and wrap in aluminum foil loosely; meat's internal temperature should reach 145 F; otherwise, air fry for 3 more minutes.
- Let it rest, then serve.

17. Mustard-Crusted Ribeye

(Ready in about 45 minutes | Serving 2|Difficulty: Medium)

Nutrition per serving: Calories 245 |Carbs 1 g| Protein 31 g |Fat 3 g

Ingredients

- Dijon mustard: 2 tsp.
- 2 ribeye steaks, (6-oz. each)

- Coarse black pepper: half tsp.

- Sea salt: 1 tsp.

Instructions

- Season steak with salt and black pepper.
- Coat the seasoned steak in mustard and let it rest on the kitchen counter for half an hour.
- Let the air fryer preheat to 390 F.
- Place steak in the oil sprayed basket of air fryer and cook for nine minutes until the steak's internal temperature reaches 140 F.
- Take it out and let it rest for five minutes, then slice and serve.

18. Burgers with Red Onion Compote

(Ready in about 40 minutes | Serving 4|Difficulty: Medium)

Nutrition per serving: Calories 398 |Carbs 14 g| Protein 33 g |Fat 12 g

Ingredients

- 2 minced cloves of garlic

- 1 and a half pounds of lean ground beef

- Sea salt: 1 tsp.

- Mayonnaise: 2 tbsp.

- Worcestershire sauce: 1 tsp.

- Black pepper: half tsp.

- Extra-virgin olive oil: 1 tsp.

- Sour cream: 2 tbsp.

- Balsamic vinegar: 1/4 cup

- Sugar: 1 tsp.

- Arugula: 1 cup

- 1 onion, cut into thin slices

- Tomato paste: 1 tbsp.

- 4 hamburger buns

Instructions

- In a bowl, add beef, one minced clove of garlic, black pepper, half tsp. salt, and Worcestershire sauce.
- Mix and make into one" thick patties. Let the patties rest for 15 minutes.
- In a pan, add oil and sauté onions for four minutes.
- Add tomato paste, sugar, and balsamic vinegar and cook for three minutes.
- Take out in a bowl and set it aside.

- Let the air fryer preheat to 350 F.
- In a bowl, add the rest of the ingredients except for buns. Mix well.
- Toast the buns and spread this mix over hamburger buns.
- Place patties in the air fryer basket and cook for six minutes, flip them and cook for 2-6 more minutes, till the internal temperature reaches 160 F.
- Take out in foil and let them rest for five minutes.
- Assemble burgers with onion compote, arugula, and patty.
- Serve right away and enjoy.

19. Keto Meatballs

(Ready in about 40 minutes | Serving 4|Difficulty: Medium)

Nutrition per serving (4 meatballs): Calories 404 |Carbs 7 g| Protein 31 g |Fat 27 g

Ingredients

- 1 pound of lean ground beef
- Grated Parmesan cheese: half cup
- 1 egg, lightly whisked
- 1 minced clove of garlic

- Mozzarella cheese, shredded: half cup
- Heavy cream: 2 tbsp.

Sauce

- Pesto: 2 tbsp.
- 1 can of tomato sauce with oregano, basil, and garlic (8 oz.)
- Heavy whipping cream: 1/4 cup

Instructions

- Let the air fryer preheat to 350 F.
- In a bowl, add all ingredients except for sauce and beef. Mix well, then add ground meat, do not over mix it.
- Make into one and a half-inch of meatballs.
- Oil spray the air fryer's basket and place meatballs inside in one even layer.
- Cook for 8 to 10 minutes until light brown and cooked through.
- In a pan, add all ingredients of the sauce, on medium flame.
- Serve meatballs with sauce.

20. Garlic & Butter Steak

(Ready in about 20 minutes | Serving 2|Difficulty: Medium)

Nutrition per serving (4 ounces): Calories 353 |Carbs 1 g| Protein 33 g |Fat 24 g

Ingredients

- One beef flat iron steak
- Minced fresh parsley: 1 tsp.
- Salt: 1/8 tsp.
- Low-sodium soy sauce: 1/4 tsp.
- Soft butter: 1 tbsp.
- Minced garlic: half tsp.
- Black pepper: 1/8 tsp.

Instructions

- Let the air fryer preheat to 400 F.
- Season the meat with salt and black pepper.
- Put steaks on a tray and inside the air fryer basket.
- Cook for 8 to 10 minutes for desired wellness. Keep checking the steak and flip halfway through.
- In a bowl, mix soy sauce, butter, garlic, and parsley.
- Serve steak with this sauce.

21. Sweet & Sour Pineapple Pork

(Ready in about 40 minutes | Serving 4|Difficulty: Medium)

Nutrition per serving: Calories 489 |Carbs 71 g| Protein 35 g |Fat 6 g

Ingredients

- 1 can of crushed pineapple, unsweetened & undrained (8 oz.)
- Sugar: half cup
- Garlic powder: 1 tsp.
- Packed dark brown sugar: half cup
- Cider vinegar: 1 cup
- Ketchup: half cup
- Low-sodium soy sauce: 2 tbsp.
- Black pepper: 1/4 tsp.
- 2 pork tenderloins, cut into halves
- Salt: 1/4 tsp.
- Dijon mustard: 1 tbsp.

Instructions

- In a pan, add pineapples and all other ingredients except for salt and black pepper.

- Let it boil, turn the heat low and let it simmer for 15 to 20 minutes until thickens. Stir often.
- Let the air fryer preheat to 350 F.
- Season the meat with salt and pepper.
- Oil spray the air fryer's basket and place meat inside.
- Cook for 7 to 8 minutes until browned edges. Flip and pour ¼ cup of sauce on pork.
- Cook 10 to 12 minutes until the internal temperature of the meat reaches 145 F.
- Let it rest for five minutes before slice and serve.
- Serve with the rest of the sauce and green onions on top.

22. Jamaican Jerk Pork Chops

(Ready in about 25 minutes | Serving 2|Difficulty: Medium)

Nutrition per serving: Calories 368 |Carbs 32 g| Protein 28 g |Fat 14 g

Ingredients

- Peach preserves: 1/4 cup
- Half of orange pepper
- 4 thin-cut, boneless pork loin chops
- Softened butter: 1 tbsp.
- Caribbean jerk seasoning: 3 tsp.

- Half of red pepper
- Salt: half tsp.
- Pepper: 1/4 tsp.
- Half of yellow pepper

Instructions

- Let the air fryer preheat to 350 F.
- In a bowl, mix peach preserves with butter and set it aside.
- Season pork chops with seasonings. Oil spray the air fryer's basket.
- Place seasoned chops in the air fryer and cook for 2 to 3 minutes on one side and then the other. Take them out and keep them warm.
- Slice the sweet peppers into thin slices.
- Cook in the air fryer, until light brown and crispy tender, for 5 to 6 minutes. Shake the basket once or twice.
- Place the steaks again in the air fryer and place butter on top.
- Cook for 1 to 2 minutes.
- Serve with peppers and rice.

23. Spiced Steaks with Cherry Sauce

(Ready in about 45 minutes | Serving 4|Difficulty: Medium)

Nutrition per serving: Calories 488 |Carbs 24 g| Protein 39 g |Fat 24 g

Ingredients

- Warmed port wine: 1/4 cup
- Dried cherries: half cup
- Kosher salt: half tsp.
- Garlic powder: 3/4 tsp.
- Paprika: 3/4 tsp.
- Brown sugar: 1 tsp.
- Ground cumin: 1/4 tsp.
- 3 and a half tsp. Roughly ground pepper
- Ground cinnamon: 1/4 tsp.
- Beef broth: 1 cup
- Ground coffee: 3/4 tsp.
- Beef tenderloin steaks: 4
- Fresh thyme, minced: 1 tsp.
- Butter: 1 tbsp.
- Heavy whipping cream: half cup
- Ground mustard: 1/8 tsp.
- 1 finely chopped shallot

Instructions

- In a bowl, mix wine and cherries.
- In another bowl, mix paprika, pepper, cinnamon, mustard, brown sugar, cumin, coffee, garlic powder, and salt. Mix well.
- Coat steaks in this spice mix. Cover them and keep them in the fridge for half an hour.
- In a skillet, add butter and sauté shallots for 2 minutes. Add thyme and broth.
- Let it boil, reduce it by half, cook for almost 8 minutes.
- Add in cream, let it boil. Cook for more 8 minutes, until it becomes thick.
- Let the air fryer preheat to 375 F.
- Oil spray the air fryer's basket and place the steak inside.
- Cook for 3 to 6 minutes on one side then the other; the internal temperature of meat should be 135 F for medium-rare and 145 F for medium-well.
- Mix cheery mix into cream mixture and serve on the side of steaks.

24. Air Fryer Steak

(Ready in about 25 minutes + 2-3 days| Serving 2|Difficulty: Medium)

Nutrition per serving: Calories 576 |Carbs 1 g| Protein 45 g |Fat 21 g

Ingredients

- 2 tbsp. of melted butter
- Strip loin steaks: 2
- 2 tsp. of black pepper
- 2 tsp. of salt

Instructions

- Season the steaks with black pepper and salt to your taste.
- Keep in the fridge for 2 to 3 days, do not cover it; keep flipping after 12 hours.
- One hour before cooking, take the steaks out of the fridge and let them rest at room temperature.
- With melted butter, brush the steak and put it in the basket of the air fryer.
- Cook for 15 minutes at 410 F. (For medium)
- Cook for 13-14 minutes for medium-rare and 16-17 minutes for well done.
- Cooking time depends upon the thickness of the steak.

25. Korean BBQ Beef

(Ready in about 45 minutes| Serving 6|Difficulty: Medium)

Nutrition per serving: Calories 487 |Carbs 32 g| Protein 39 g |Fat 22 g

Ingredients

- Corn Starch: 1/4 Cup
- 1 Pound of Flank Steak, cut into thin slices

Sauce

- White Wine Vinegar: 2 tbsp.
- Soy Sauce: half cup
- Water: 1 tbsp.
- Brown Sugar: half cup
- 1 minced clove of garlic
- Ground Ginger: 1 tsp.
- Cornstarch: 1 tbsp.
- Sesame Seeds: half tsp.
- Hot Chili Sauce: 1 tbsp.

Instructions

- Coat the thinly cut steak in the cornstarch.
- Oil spray the air fryer's basket
- Spray the coated steak with oil and place it in the basket.
- Cook at 390 F for ten minutes. Flip and cook for ten more minutes.

- In a pan, add all ingredients of sauce except for cornstarch.
- Let it boil on low flame and add in water and cornstarch mixture.
- Coat the cooked steak in the sauce.
- Serve with sautéed vegetables and rice.

26. Ham & Cheese Turnovers

(Ready in about 30 minutes| Serving 4|Difficulty: Medium)

Nutrition per serving: Calories 357 |Carbs 55 g| Protein 15 g |Fat 10 g

Ingredients

- Black forest deli ham, cut into thin slices: 1/4 pound
- Crumbled blue cheese: 2 tbsp.
- 1 pear, cut into thin slices
- 1 (13.8 oz.) pizza crust, refrigerated
- Toasted chopped walnuts: 1/4 cup

Instructions

- Let the air fryer preheat to 400 F.
- Cut pizza crust into 12" square and slice into four parts.

- In each part, diagonally add blue cheese, half pear slices, walnuts, and ham. Fold like a triangle. Seal the edges with a fork.
- Oil spray the air fryer's basket and place turnover inside and cook for 4 to 6 minutes,
- On one side and then flip.
- Serve warm and enjoy.

27. Raspberry Balsamic Pork Chops

(Ready in about 30 minutes| Serving 4|Difficulty: Medium)

Nutrition per serving: Calories 579 |Carbs 36 g| Protein 32 g |Fat 36 g

Ingredients

- 4 bone-in smoked pork chops
- Balsamic vinegar: 1/3 cup
- Milk: 1/4 cup
- Bread crumbs: 1 cup
- 2 eggs
- Chopped pecans: 1 cup
- Brown sugar: 2 tbsp.
- Concentrate orange juice: 1 tbsp.
- All-purpose flour: 1/4 of cup
- Raspberry jam, seedless: 2 tbsp.

Instructions

- Let the air fryer preheat to 400 F.
- In a bowl, mix milk and eggs.
- In a separate bowl, mix pecans with bread crumbs.
- Coat the chops in flour, then in the egg mix, and lastly in pecan mix.
- Oil spray the air fryer's basket and place pork chops inside in one even layer and spray with oil.
- Cook for 12 to 15 minutes until the meat's internal temperature reaches 145 F. Flip the chops halfway through.
- In a pan, add the rest of the ingredients and let them boil, until thickens, for 6 to 8 minutes.
- Serve right away with sauce and enjoy.

28. Nacho Hot Dogs

(Ready in about 35 minutes| Serving 6|Difficulty: Medium)

Nutrition per serving: Calories 216 |Carbs 26 g| Protein 9 g |Fat 9 g

Ingredients

- Crushed tortilla chips nacho-flavored: 1 cup
- Cheddar cheese sticks: 3, cut in half lengthwise
- Self-rising flour: 1 and 1/4 cups

- Chili powder: 1/4 tsp.
- Plain Greek yogurt: 1 cup
- Hot dogs: 6
- Chopped jalapeno: 3 tbsp. Without seeds
- Salsa: 1/4 cup

Instructions

- Make a slit in hot dogs. Do not completely cut them, and place a cheese stick in the slit.
- Let the air fryer preheat to 350 F.
- In a bowl, mix yogurt, jalapenos, flour, tortilla chips (1/4 cup), salsa, and chili powder, make into a soft dough.
- Divide dough into six parts and roll into 15" strips.
- Wrap around the cheese-hot dog. Wrap all the hot dogs and spray with oil, and coat in crushed chips.
- Oil spray the air fryer's basket and place hot dogs inside in one even layer.
- Cook for 8 to 10 minutes until lightly browned, and cheese is melty.
- Serve with guacamole and sour cream.

Chapter 6: Air-Fry Seafood Recipes

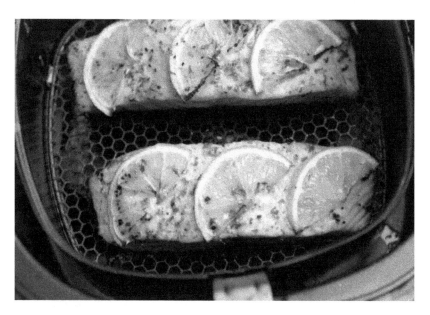

1. Fish & Fries

(Ready in about 35 minutes| Serving 4|Difficulty: Medium)

Nutrition per serving: Calories 143 |Carbs 18 g| Protein 21 g |Fat 6 g

Ingredients

- Pepper: 1/4 tsp.
- 2 medium potatoes
- Salt: 1/4 tsp.
- Olive oil: 2 tbsp.

For Fish

- 1 pound of cod fillets
- Crushed cornflakes: 2/3 cup
- All-purpose flour: 1/3 cup
- Parmesan cheese, grated: 1 tbsp.
- Pepper: 1/4 tsp.
- 1 egg
- Water: 2 tbsp.
- Cayenne pepper: 1/8 tsp.
- Salt: ¼ tsp.

Instructions

- Let the air fryer preheat to 400 F.
- Cut the peeled potatoes in half" thick slices, then cut into sticks.
- In a bowl, add oil, salt, fries, and pepper. Toss it well.
- Place in the air fryer in one even layer cook for 5 to 10 minutes, shake the basket and cook for 5 to 10 minutes more.
- In a bowl, mix pepper and flour.
- In another bowl, mix water with egg.
- In the third bowl, mix cornflakes with cayenne and cheese.
- Season fish fillets with salt and coat in the flour mix, then in the egg mixture, and lastly in cornflakes mix.

- Take fries out and keep them warm.
- Place fillets in the air fryer in one even layer and cook for 8 to 10 minutes, until fork-tender.
- Carefully flip halfway through cooking.
- Serve fish with fries, and enjoy.

2. Salmon & Brussels Sprouts

(Ready in about 15 minutes| Serving 4|Difficulty: Medium)

Nutrition per serving: Calories 187 |Carbs 2 g| Protein 25 g |Fat 3 g

Ingredients

- 4 fillets of salmon
- Fresh thyme leaves, chopped: 1 tsp.
- 4 cloves of minced garlic
- Olive oil: 2 tbsp.
- Kosher salt: 2 tsp.
- Black pepper: 1 tsp.
- Honey: 1 tbsp.
- 1 pound of Brussels sprouts
- Balsamic vinegar: 1 tbsp.

Instructions

- In a bowl, add half of the minced garlic.

- In another bowl, add the rest of the minced garlic, olive oil, kosher salt (1 tsp.), thyme leaves (1 tsp.), the juice from lemon, black pepper (half tsp.). Mix it well and brush the fish fillets with this mixture.
- Let the air fryer preheat to 400 F.
- Oil spray the air fryer's basket.
- Put fish in the air fryer, skin side down in the last rack. Leave some space in fillets.
- In a bowl, add olive oil (1 tbsp.), salt (1 tsp.), remaining garlic, black pepper (half tsp.) mix it well.
- Cut the Brussel sprouts in half, add the remaining garlic bowl and toss well.
- Put in the above rack of air fryer and cook for 6 to 8 minutes.
- Take salmon out and keep air frying sprouts for 1 to 3 more minutes.
- In a bowl, add the rest of the ingredients and mix.
- Pour over salmon and sprouts and serve.

3. Air Fryer Easy Salmon

(Ready in about 15 minutes| Serving 2|Difficulty: Easy)

Nutrition per serving: Calories 134 |Carbs 3 g| Protein 25 g |Fat 2 g

Ingredients

- Olive oil: 2 tsp.

- 2 salmon fillets

- 1 minced clove of garlic

- Black pepper, to taste

- Thyme leaves: half tsp.
- Whole grain mustard: 2 tbsp.

- Kosher salt, to taste

- Packed brown sugar: 1 tbsp.

Instructions

- Sprinkle salt and black pepper on salmon. In a bowl, add thyme, oil, garlic, mustard, and sugar, mix well and brush over salmon.
- Place fish in the air fryer basket and cook for ten minutes at 400 F.
- Serve and enjoy.

4. Bacon Wrapped Scallops

(Ready in about 15 minutes| Serving 4|Difficulty: Easy)

Nutrition per serving: Calories 198 |Carbs 9 g| Protein 24 g |Fat 9 g

Ingredients

- BBQ Sauce: 1/4 cup
- 8 center-cut bacon slices
- 16 sea scallops (large)

Instructions

- Cut bacon in half, and air fry them for 3 minutes at 400 F.
- Dry the scallops well.
- With bacon slices, wrap the scallops and seal with toothpicks.
- Put them in the air fryer in one even layer.
- Brush the wrapped scallops with BBQ sauce. Or spray with oil and black pepper, and salt.
- Air fry for five minutes at 400 F. flip them and brush with sauce again and cook for 5 more minutes.
- Serve right away.

5. Air Fryer Cajun Shrimp

(Ready in about 30 minutes| Serving 4|Difficulty: Medium)

Nutrition per serving: Calories 215|Carbs 3 g| Protein 26 g |Fat 9 g

Ingredients

- 24 peeled shrimp (extra jumbo)
- Cajun seasoning: 1 tbsp.

- 1 zucchini, cut into half-moons (¼" thick)
- Olive oil: 2 tbsp.
- 1 yellow squash, cut into half-moons (¼" thick)
- Kosher salt: ¼ tsp.
- 6 oz. of cooked chicken sausage, cut into slices
- 1 red bell pepper, cut without seeds into 1" pieces

Instructions

- In a bowl, add shrimps and Cajun seasoning, coat them well.
- In a bowl, add vegetables, oil, and sausage and mix to combine.
- Let the air fryer preheat to 400 F.
- In the air fryer basket, add shrimps and vegetable mix in one even layer.
- Cook for 8 minutes, and after 2-3 minutes, shake the basket.
- Serve right away.

6. Tortilla Crusted Tilapia Salad

(Ready in about 15 minutes| Serving 2|Difficulty: Easy)

Nutrition per serving: Calories 234|Carbs 3 g| Protein 27 g |Fat 7 g

Ingredients

- Chipotle lime dressing: half cup
- 6 cups of mixed greens
- 1/3 cup of chopped red onion
- 1 cup of cherry tomatoes
- 2 Tilapia fillets (tortilla crusted)

Instructions

- Oil spray the fish fillets on every side.
- Put in the basket of air fryer and cook for 15 to 18 minutes at 390 F.
- In two bowls, mix half of all vegetables, pour over the lime dressing.
- Put fish fillet on top and serve right away.

7. Air-Fryer Scallops

(Ready in about 25 minutes| Serving 2|Difficulty: Medium)

Nutrition per serving: Calories 298 |Carbs 33 g| Protein 28 g |Fat 5 g

Ingredients

- 6 sea scallops
- 1 egg
- All-purpose flour: 2 tbsp.
- Mashed potato flakes: 1/3 cup

- Salt: 1/8 tsp.
- Bread crumbs, seasoned: 1/3 cup
- Pepper: 1/8 tsp.

Instructions

- Let the air fryer preheat to 400 F.
- In a bowl, add whisked egg.
- In a separate bowl, add bread crumbs, pepper, potato flakes, and salt.
- In a bowl, add flour and scallops (dry them well), toss them to coat.
- Then coat in egg and lastly in potato mix.
- Oil spray the air fryer's basket put scallops in the basket, and spray them with oil. Cook for 3 to 4 minutes' flip and cook for 3 to 4 minutes more.

8. Salmon with Maple-Dijon Glaze

(Ready in about 35 minutes| Serving 4|Difficulty: Medium)

Nutrition per serving: Calories 329 |Carbs 11 g| Protein 19 g |Fat 23 g

Ingredients

- 4 salmon fillets
- Butter: 3 tbsp.
- Dijon mustard: 1 tbsp.

- Maple syrup: 3 tbsp.
- Juice of one lemon
- Olive oil: 1 tbsp.
- 1 minced clove to garlic
- Salt: 1/4 tsp.
- Pepper: 1/4 tsp.

Instructions

- Let the air fryer preheat to 400 F.
- In a pan, add butter on medium flame, add minced garlic, maple syrup, lemon juice, and mustard.
- Turn heat to low and cook for 2 to 3 minutes, until it becomes thick. Turn off the heat and set it aside.
- Coat the fish fillets in salt, oil, and pepper.
- Put salmon in the basket of the air fryer. Cook for 5 to 7 minutes, until it is fork-tender.
- Pour sauce over and serve.

9. Crumbed Fish

(Ready in about 22 minutes| Serving 4|Difficulty: Medium)

Nutrition per serving: Calories 354 |Carbs 22 g| Protein 27 g |Fat 17 g

Ingredient

- Flounder fillets: 4

- Dry bread crumbs: 1 cup
- 1 lemon, cut into slices
- Vegetable oil: ¼ cup
- 1 egg, whisked

Instructions

- Let the air fryer preheat to 350 F.
- In a bowl, mix oil and crumbs well.
- Coat fish fillets in egg then in bread crumbs.
- In the basket of the air fryer, place breaded fish.
- Cook for 12 minutes, until fork-tender.
- Serve with lemon slices on top.

10. Cajun Air Fryer Salmon

(Ready in about 20 minutes| Serving 2|Difficulty: Medium)

Nutrition per serving: Calories 327|Carbs 4 g| Protein 33 g |Fat 18 g

Ingredients

- Brown sugar: 1 tsp.
- 2 skin-on fillets of salmon
- Cajun seasoning: 1 tbsp.

Instructions

- Let the air fryer preheat to 390 F.

- Clean and dry the fish with a paper towel. Oil spray the fish, and in a bowl, mix sugar and Cajun seasoning, sprinkle over fish, and coat well.
- Oil spray the air fryer's basket and place fish in the basket of the air fryer.
- Lightly spray the fish with oil.
- Cook at 390 F for 8 minutes.
- Serve right away and enjoy.

11. Crab Cakes

(Ready in about 1 hour & 25 minutes| Serving 4|Difficulty: Medium)

Nutrition per serving: Calories 242|Carbs 10 g| Protein 28 g |Fat 9 g

Ingredient

- Mayonnaise: 2 tbsp.
- 1 egg, whisked
- Worcestershire sauce: 1 tsp.
- Seafood seasoning: 1 tsp.
- Dijon mustard: 1 tsp.
- Hot pepper sauce: half tsp.
- Baking powder: 1 tsp.
- 1 pound of lump crabmeat

- Chopped green onion: 2 tbsp.
- Salt & black pepper, to taste
- Milk: 3 tbsp.
- 11 crushed saltine crackers

Instructions

- In a bowl, mix mustard, mayonnaise, green onion, hot pepper sauce, egg, seafood seasoning, and Worcestershire sauce. Mix well and set it aside.
- In a bowl, add crab meat, break with a spoon.
- Add pepper, milk, and salt, mix well.
- Add baking powder and crushed crackers and mix lightly.
- Add into the egg mix, mix carefully.
- Shape into eight patties. Keep in the fridge for 1-8 hours.
- Let the air fryer preheat to 400 F.
- Oil spray the crab cakes and place them in the basket of the air fryer.
- Cook at 400 F for five minutes, flip the cakes and cook for five more minutes.

12. Salmon Cakes with Sriracha Mayo

(Ready in about 40 minutes| Serving 4|Difficulty: Medium)

Nutrition per serving: Calories 340|Carbs 4 g| Protein 25 g |Fat 24 g

Ingredients

Sriracha Mayo

- Sriracha: 1 tbsp.
- Mayonnaise: ¼ cup

Salmon Cakes

- 1 and a half tsp. of seafood seasoning
- 1 pound of salmon skinless fillets, slice into one" pieces
- 1 egg, whisked lightly
- Almond flour: ⅓ cup
- 1 chopped green onion

Instructions

- In a bowl, mix Sriracha and mayonnaise.
- In a food processor, add one tbsp. of Sriracha mayo, green onion, almond flour, seafood seasoning, egg, and salmon. Pulse 4-5 times until combined. Do not over mix.
- Make into eight patties and keep in the fridge for 15 minutes.
- Let the air fryer preheat to 390 F.
- Oil spray the air fryer's basket.

- Spray the patties with oil and place them in the air fryer in one even layer.
- Cook for 6-8 minutes.
- Serve right away with spicy mayo.

13. Lemon Pepper Shrimp

(Ready in about 15 minutes| Serving 2|Difficulty: Easy)

Nutrition per serving: Calories 215|Carbs 12 g| Protein 28 g |Fat 8 g

Ingredients

- 12 oz. of raw medium peeled shrimp, deveined
- Juice and slice of one lemon
- Olive oil: 1 tbsp.
- Paprika: ¼ tsp.
- Lemon pepper: 1 tsp.
- Garlic powder: ¼ tsp.

Instructions

- Let the air fryer preheat to 400 F.
- In a bowl, mix all ingredients except for shrimps and lemon slices. Mix well and add shrimps and toss to combine.
- Put seasoned shrimps in the basket of air fryer and cook for 6-8 minutes.

- Serve lemon slices on the side of shrimps.

14. Lobster Tails with Lemon-Garlic Butter

(Ready in about 20 minutes| Serving 2|Difficulty: Easy)

Nutrition per serving: Calories 313|Carbs 4 g| Protein 18 g |Fat 25 g

Ingredients

- Butter: 4 tbsp.
- 2 lobster tails
- Lemon zest: 1 tsp.
- Lemon wedges: 2
- 1 minced clove of garlic
- Fresh parsley, chopped: 1 tsp.
- Salt & black pepper, to taste

Instructions

- Make the lobster butterfly style with a sharp knife. Spread the halves of the tail.
- In a pan, melt butter, adds garlic and zest, cook for 30 seconds.
- Brush the tail with 2 tbsp. of garlic butter.
- Put the lobster in the air fryer's basket; make sure the meat will be face up.
- Season it with black pepper and salt.

- Air fry for 5-7 minutes, at 380 F.
- Pour over the lobster with the remaining butter.
- Serve tails with lemon wedges and parsley on top.

15. Shrimp & Polenta

(Ready in about 45 minutes| Serving 2|Difficulty: Medium)

Nutrition per serving: Calories 333|Carbs 12 g| Protein 22 g |Fat 19 g

Ingredients

- Olive oil: 2 tsp.
- Grape tomatoes: 12
- Half tube of polenta, cut into six rounds
- 8 oz. of jumbo peeled shrimp, deveined
- Hot pepper sauce: 1 tsp.
- Salt & black pepper, to taste
- Softened unsalted butter: 2 tbsp.
- Lemon-pepper seasoning: half tsp.
- Chopped fresh parsley: 2 tsp.

Instructions

- Let the air fryer preheat to 400 F.
- Place polenta circles on a flat surface and brush with one tsp. of olive oil on both sides.

- Season with black pepper and salt.
- In a bowl, add tomatoes and shrimps. Add one tsp. of olive oil and toss to combine.
- Place tomatoes in the air fryer basket and cook for 2 minutes. Take them out and smash them.
- Put shrimps in the air fryer basket and cook for ten minutes. Take them out in the tomatoes
- Put polenta in the air fryer basket and let it cook for 15 minutes, turn the pieces and cook for 15 more minutes.
- In a bowl, add the rest of the ingredients and mix well.
- On two plates, take polenta out and add shrimp tomatoes on top, and drizzle over the butter sauce.

16. Shrimp Bang Bang

(Ready in about 39 minutes| Serving 4|Difficulty: Medium)

Nutrition per serving: Calories 415|Carbs 32 g| Protein 23 g |Fat 23 g

Ingredients

- 1 pound of uncooked peeled shrimp, deveined
- Mayonnaise: half cup
- Sriracha sauce: 1 tbsp.
- 1 head of lettuce leaves
- All-purpose flour: ¼ cup

- Sweet chili sauce: ¼ cup
- Panko bread crumbs: 1 cup
- 2 chopped green onions

Instructions

- Let the air fryer preheat to 400 F
- In a bowl, mix sriracha sauce, mayonnaise, and chili sauce. Take some sauce out for dipping.
- In two different bowls, add flour and panko.
- Cover shrimps in flour, then in mayo sauce, and lastly in panko.
- Put breaded shrimps in the basket of the air fryer in one even layer.
- Cook at 400 F for 12 minutes.
- In lettuce leaves, place the cooked shrimps and serve with sauce.

17. Salmon Nuggets

(Ready in about 35 minutes| Serving 4|Difficulty: Medium)

Nutrition per serving: Calories 364|Carbs 27 g| Protein 25 g |Fat 16 g

Ingredients

- 1 center-cut, skinless, salmon fillet, slice into 1 and a half" of pieces

- Maple syrup: ⅓ cup
- Sea salt, one pinch
- Dried ground chipotle pepper: ¼ teaspoon
- 1 and a half cups of butter
- 1 egg
- Croutons: garlic-flavored, as needed

Instructions

- In a pan, add chipotle powder, salt, and maple syrup. Mix and let it boil over medium flame. Turn the heat very low.
- In a food processor, add croutons, and make them into crumbs. Take out in a bowl.
- In a separate bowl, add whisked egg.
- Let the air fryer preheat to 390 F.
- Season salmon with salt.
- Coat salmon in egg then in croutons.
- Place on a baking dish and spray with oil.
- Oil spray the air fryer's basket, place fish nuggets inside in one even layer, and cook for three minutes.
- Flip the nuggets and spray with oil and cook for 3-4 minutes.
- Serve with maple sauce.

18. Fish Sticks

(Ready in about 20 minutes| Serving 4|Difficulty: Medium)

Nutrition per serving: Calories 200|Carbs 16 g| Protein 25 g |Fat 4 g

Ingredients

- All-purpose flour: ¼ cup

- Grated parmesan cheese: ¼ cup

- 1 pound of cod fillets

- 1 whole egg

- Paprika: 1 tsp.

- Panko bread crumbs: half cup

- Black pepper, to taste

- Parsley flakes: 1 tbsp.

Instructions

- Let the air fryer preheat to 400 F.
- Slice the fillet into fish sticks.
- In a bowl, add flour; in another bowl, add whisked egg.
- In a separate bowl, add pepper, panko, paprika, Parmesan cheese, and parsley.

- Dip cod sticks in flour, second in the whisked egg, and lastly in panko mix. Oil spray the air fryer's basket.
- Place breaded sticks in the air fryer basket in one even layer and spray them with oil spray.
- Cook for five minutes, flip and cook for five more minutes.

19. Crispy Fish Po' Boys

(Ready in about 20 minutes| Serving 4|Difficulty: Medium)

Nutrition per serving: Calories 321|Carbs 45 g| Protein 35 g |Fat 31 g

Ingredients

Fish

- Panko bread crumbs: half cup
- All-purpose flour: ¼ cup
- 4 fillets of white fish
- Black pepper: half tsp.
- 1 tbsp. of water
- Salt: ¼ tsp.
- Garlic powder: ¼ tsp.
- Cornmeal: ¼ cup
- 1 large egg

Slaw

- Dried ground chipotle pepper: ¼ teaspoon
- Sour cream: ⅓ cup
- Fresh chopped cilantro: ¼ cup
- Lime juice: 1 tbsp.
- Shredded carrot with cabbage: 3 cups
- Salt: ¼ tsp.
- Mayonnaise: ¼ cup

Instructions

- Oil spray the air fryer's basket.
- In a dish, add salt, flour, garlic powder, and black pepper mix well.
- In another bowl, mix the whisked egg with water.
- In a separate bowl, mix cornmeal and bread crumbs.
- Coat fish in flour, then in egg, and lastly in crumbs mix.
- Spray the fish with oil and place it in the air fryer in one even layer.
- Cook for 6-10 minutes at 400 F, until fork tender.
- In a bowl, mix chipotle pepper, mayonnaise, salt, sour cream, and lime juice.
- Add the shredded vegetable and cilantro and mix.

- In the bread rolls, serve fish with chipotle slaw and lime wedges.

20. Honey Pecan Shrimp

(Ready in about 35 minutes| Serving 4|Difficulty: Medium)

Nutrition per serving: Calories 334|Carbs 8 g| Protein 31 g |Fat 9 g

Ingredients

- 1 pound of uncooked peeled shrimps, deveined
- Cornstarch: 1/4 cup
- Pepper: 1/4 tsp.
- Sea salt: 3/4 tsp.
- Chopped pecans: 2/3 cup
- Honey: 1/4 cup
- 2 whites from egg
- Mayonnaise: 2 tbsp.

Instructions

- In a bowl, mix salt (half tsp.), pepper, and cornstarch.
- In another bowl, whisk the whites till foamy and soft.
- In a separate bowl, add remaining salt and pecans.

- Coat the shrimps in cornstarch, secondly in whites, and lastly in pecan mix.

- Let the air fryer preheat to 330 F.

- Place shrimps in the basket of air fryer and spray with oil, cook for five minutes.

- Flip and cook for five more minutes.

- In a bowl, mix mayonnaise and honey mix well.

- Take the cooked shrimp in the honey sauce toss well.

- Serve right away.

21. Pecan-Crusted Tilapia

(Ready in about 15 minutes| Serving 4|Difficulty: Easy)

Nutrition per serving: Calories 314|Carbs 4 g| Protein 21 g |Fat 9 g

Ingredients

- 1 pound of boneless and skinless tilapia filets

- Melted butter: 1/4 cup

- Paprika: 1/4 tsp.

- Chopped pecans: 1 cup

- Lemon wedges: 4-5

- Dried rosemary: 1 tsp.

- Sea salt: 1 tsp.

- Chopped parsley: 2 tbsp.

Instructions

- Coat the fish in melted butter.

- In a bowl, mix paprika, salt, pecans, and rosemary.

- Let the air fryer preheat to 350 F.

- Put the fish fillet in the basket of air fryer and sprinkle generously with pecan mix.

- Air fry for 6-8 minutes.

- Take the fish out and serve with lemon wedges and parsley on top.

22. Maple-Crusted Salmon

(Ready in about 45 minutes| Serving 2|Difficulty: Medium)

Nutrition per serving: Calories 334|Carbs 7 g| Protein 21 g |Fat 9 g

Ingredients

- Finely chopped walnuts: half cup

- 12 oz. Of salmon filets

- Worcestershire sauce: 1 tsp.

- Dijon mustard: 2 tsp.

- Half lemon

- Maple syrup: 1/3 cup

- Sea salt: half tsp.

Instructions

- Coat the salmon with mustard, maple syrup, and Worcestershire sauce.

- Keep in the fridge for half an hour.

- Let the air fryer preheat to 350 F.

- Take fish out of the sauce and coat with chopped nuts, and sprinkle with salt.

- Place fish in the air fryer basket and cook for 6-8 minutes till fish is fork-tender.

- Serve the fish with parsley on top.

23. Beer-Breaded Halibut Fish Tacos

(Ready in about 45 minutes| Serving 4|Difficulty: Medium)

Ingredients

- 1 pound of halibut, slice into one" of strips

- Greek yogurt: 1/4 cup

- Light beer: 1 cup

- 1 minced clove of garlic

- 1 finely chopped jalapeño

- Ground cumin: 1/4 tsp.

- All-purpose flour: 1/4 cup

- 1 + 1/4 tsp. sea salt

- Cornmeal: half cup

- Chopped onion: 1/4 cup

- Juice form one lime

- Mayonnaise: 1/4 cup

- Shredded cabbage: 2 cups

- Grape tomatoes: 1 cup, cut into quarters

- Corn tortillas: 8

- Chopped cilantro: half cup

- 1 whisked egg

Instructions

- In a bowl, mix cumin, beer, jalapeno (1 tsp.), garlic, and the fish. Mix well and keep in the fridge for half an hour.
- In a bowl, mix flour, salt (half tsp.), and cornmeal.
- In another bowl, mix lime juice (1 tbsp.), salt (half tsp.), mayonnaise, cabbage, and yogurt.
- In a bowl, mix the rest of the jalapeño, tomatoes, salt (1/4 tsp.), onion, lime juice, and cilantro mix well; Pico de Gallo is ready.
- Take the fish out and coat in egg and then in cornmeal mix.
- Let the air fryer preheat to 350 F.
- Spray the fish with oil and cook for six minutes; flip and cook for four more minutes.
- Warm the tortillas.
- Put air-fried fish in a warmed tortilla with Pico de Gallo and slaw.
- Serve right away.

24. Catfish & Green Beans

(Ready in about 25 minutes| Serving 2|Difficulty: Medium)

Nutrition per serving: Calories 416|Carbs 31 g| Protein 33 g |Fat 18 g

Ingredients

- Light brown sugar: 1 tsp.
- Fresh green beans: 1 and a half cups, trimmed
- Kosher salt, to taste
- 2 catfish fillets
- Crushed red pepper: half tsp.
- Mayonnaise: 2 tbsp.
- 1 egg, whisked
- Panko bread crumbs: ⅓ cup
- All-purpose flour: ¼ cup
- Apple cider vinegar: half tsp.
- Black pepper: ¼ tsp.
- Fresh dill: 1 and a half tsp.
- Granulated sugar: ⅛ teaspoon
- Dill pickle relish: ¾ teaspoon

Instructions

- In a bowl, add green beans and spray generously with oil.

- Season with crushed red pepper, salt (1/8 tsp.), and brown sugar. Toss and place in the basket of air fryer and cook for 12 minutes at 400 F.

- Coat the fish in flour, then dip in egg, and lastly coat in panko.

- Spray oil the fish fillet and place it in the basket of the air fryer.

- Cook for 8 minutes at 400 F.

- Season with salt (1/4 tsp) and black pepper.

- In a bowl, mix relish, sugar, dill, mayo, and vinegar.

- Serve the catfish with lemon slices and sauces.

25. Popcorn Shrimp

(Ready in about 30 minutes| Serving 4|Difficulty: Medium)

Nutrition per serving: Calories 297|Carbs 35 g| Protein 29 g |Fat 4 g

Ingredients

- Garlic powder: 1 tbsp.
- 2 eggs, whisked
- Water: 2 tbsp.
- All-purpose flour: half cup
- 1 pound of small peeled shrimp, deveined
- Ground cumin: 1 tbsp.
- Ketchup: half cup
- Fresh cilantro, chopped: 2 tablespoons
- Panko breadcrumbs: 1 and a half cups
- Lime juice: 2 tbsp.

- Chipotle chilies chopped: 2 tbsp. (in adobo)
- Kosher salt: ⅛ tsp.

Instructions

- Oil spray the air fryer's basket.
- In a bowl, add flour.
- In another bowl, mix water with eggs.
- In a third bowl, mix garlic powder, panko, and cumin.
- Coat shrimps in flour, secondly in egg, and lastly in panko.
- Put shrimps in the basket of air fryer and spray with oil.
- Cook for 8 minutes at 360 F, flipping halfway through cooking.
- In a bowl, mix the rest of the ingredients and serve with shrimps.

26. Scallops with Lemon-Herb Sauce

(Ready in about 20 minutes| Serving 2|Difficulty: Medium)

Nutrition per serving: Calories 348|Carbs 5 g| Protein 14 g |Fat 30 g

Ingredients

- Finely grated lemon zest: 1 tsp.
- Black pepper: ¼ teaspoon

- Salt: ⅛ teaspoon
- 8 sea scallops, large
- Capers: 2 tsp., chopped
- Olive oil: ¼ cup
- Minced garlic: half tsp.
- Flat-leaf parsley, chopped: 2 tbsp.

Instructions

- Season scallops with salt and black pepper.

- Oil spray the air fryer's basket.

- Put seasoned scallops in the air fryer basket.

- Cook for six minutes, at 400°F.

- In a bowl, mix the rest of the ingredients.

- Pour over scallops and serve.

27. Gingered Honey Salmon

(Ready in about 20 minutes| Serving 6|Difficulty: Medium)

Nutrition per serving: Calories 237|Carbs 15 g| Protein 20 g |Fat 10 g

Ingredients

- 1 salmon fillet
- Orange juice: 1/3 cup

- Honey: 1/4 cup
- Garlic powder: 1 tsp.
- 1 chopped green onion
- Soy sauce: 1/3 cup
- Ground ginger: 1 tsp.

Instructions

- In a bowl, add all ingredients except for salmon. Mix well, and take 2/3 cup out in a bowl, add salmon, and coat the fish well.
- Keep in the fridge for half an hour.
- Let the air fryer preheat to 325 F.
- Oil spray the air fryer's basket and place the fish inside and cook for 15 to 18 minutes.
- Keep basting with the remaining marinade in the last five minutes of cooking.

28. Salmon with Horseradish Rub

(Ready in about 30 minutes| Serving 2|Difficulty: Medium)

Nutrition per serving: Calories 305|Carbs 7 g| Protein 35 g |Fat 15 g

Ingredients

- Capers: 1 tbsp. Finely diced
- Salt & black pepper: ¼ tsp. Of each

- Grated horseradish: 2 tbsp.
- Olive oil: 1 tbsp.
- 1 skinless salmon fillet
- Chopped flat-leaf parsley: 2 tbsp.

Instructions

- Oil spray the air fryer's basket.
- In a bowl, mix parsley, oil, horseradish, and capers.
- Season the salmon with black pepper and salt.
- Coat the salmon with horseradish mix and oil spray the fish.
- Air fry the fish at 375 F for 15 minutes or until the internal temperature reaches 130 F.
- Serve right away.

29. Fish Cakes

(Ready in about 20 minutes| Serving 2|Difficulty: Medium)

Nutrition per serving: Calories 399|Carbs 28 g| Protein 35 g |Fat 16 g

Ingredients

- 10 oz. of chopped white fish
- Salt: ⅛ teaspoon
- Black pepper, to taste
- Thai sweet chili sauce: 2 tbsp.

- 1 egg
- Panko breadcrumbs: 2/3 cup
- Fresh cilantro, chopped: 3 tbsp.
- Mayonnaise: 2 tbsp.

Instructions

- Oil spray the air fryer's basket
- In a bowl, mix all seasonings and chopped fish; mix well but do not overmix.
- Make into 4 patties, and spray with oil.
- Place in the air fryer and cook for 9-10 minutes at 400 F.
- Serve with your favorite dipping sauce.

30. Mahi Mahi with Brown Butter

(Ready in about 20 minutes| Serving 4|Difficulty: Easy)

Nutrition per serving: Calories 416|Carbs 12 g| Protein 31 g |Fat 31 g

Ingredients

- 4 Mahi Mahi fillets
- Butter: ⅔ cup
- Salt & black pepper, to taste

Instructions

- Let the air fryer preheat to 350 F.
- Season the fish with black pepper and salt.
- Oil spray the seasoned fish.
- Place the fish in the basket of the air fryer in one even layer.
- Cook for 12 minutes until fork tender.
- In a pan, add butter on medium flame and melt and let it simmer for 3-5 minutes until it turns dark brown and frothy, do not burn the burn.
- Drizzle over air-fried fish and serve.

31. Coconut Shrimp

(Ready in about 45 minutes| Serving 6|Difficulty: Medium)

Nutrition per serving: Calories 236|Carbs 27 g| Protein 14 g |Fat 9 g

Ingredients

- 2 eggs
- Flaked coconut, unsweetened: ⅔ cup
- All-purpose flour: half cup
- Panko bread crumbs: ⅓ cup
- 12 oz. Of raw peeled shrimp, deveined

- Kosher salt: half tsp.
- 1 serrano chili, cut into thin slices
- Ground black pepper: 1 and a half tsp.
- Honey: ¼ cup
- Fresh cilantro chopped: 2 tbsp.
- Lime juice: ¼ cup

Instructions

- In a bowl, mix pepper and flour.
- In another bowl, whisk the eggs.
- In a separate bowl, mix panko and coconut flakes.
- Coat shrimps in flour, then in egg, and lastly in panko mix.
- Spray the breaded shrimps with oil.
- Let the air fryer preheat to 400 F.
- Put breaded shrimps in the basket of air fryer cook for three minutes.
- Flip and cook for 3 more minutes.
- Season with salt.
- In a bowl, mix serrano chili, lime juice, and honey.
- Serve shrimps with honey dip.

32. Spicy Bay Scallops

(Ready in about 15 minutes| Serving 4|Difficulty: Easy)

Nutrition per serving: Calories 179|Carbs 7 g| Protein 28 g |Fat 4 g

Ingredients

- 1 pound of bay scallops, cleaned
- Olive oil: 2 tsp.
- Smoked paprika: 2 tsp.
- Cayenne red pepper: 1/8 tsp.
- Chili powder: 2 tsp.
- Garlic powder: 1 tsp.
- Black pepper: ¼ tsp.

Instructions

- Let the air fryer preheat to 400 F.
- In a bowl, add all ingredients and toss well.
- Put in the basket of the air fryer.
- Cook for 8 minutes, shake the basket after 4 minutes, and cook for 4 more minutes.

Chapter 7: Air-Fry Vegetables & Sides Recipes

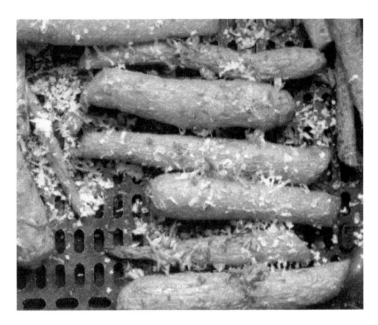

1. Fried Avocado Tacos

(Ready in about 40 minutes| Serving 4|Difficulty: Medium)

Nutrition per serving: Calories 407|Carbs 48 g| Protein 9 g |Fat 21 g

Ingredients

- Fresh cilantro minced: 1/4 cup
- Coleslaw mix: 2 cups
- Honey: 1 tsp.
- Salt: 1/4 tsp.

- Pepper: 1/4 tsp.
- 1 egg, whisked
- Ground chipotle pepper: 1/4 tsp.
- 2 peeled avocados, sliced
- Plain Greek yogurt: 1/4 cup
- Lime juice: 2 tbsp.
- Cornmeal: 1/4 cup
- Salt: half tsp.
- Garlic powder: half tsp.
- 1 chopped tomato
- Ground chipotle pepper: half tsp.
- 8 tortillas (6")

Instructions

- Let the air fryer preheat to 400 F.
- In a bowl, add the egg.
- In a separate bowl, mix garlic powder, chipotle pepper, salt, and cornmeal.
- Coat slices of avocado in the egg after that in the cornmeal mix.
- In a large bowl, add the rest of the ingredients, except for the tortilla, tomato, mix well and keep in the fridge.
- Oil spray the air fryer's basket.

- Place breaded avocado slices in the air fryer basket in one even layer.
- Cook for four minutes' flip and spray with oil and cook for 3 to 4 more minutes until golden brown.
- Put avocado slices in a tortilla with coleslaw mix and tomatoes.
- Serve right away.

2. Baked Potatoes

(Ready in about 55 minutes| Serving 2|Difficulty: Medium)

Nutrition per serving: Calories 407|Carbs 48 g| Protein 9 g |Fat 21 g

Ingredients

- 1 tsp. neutral oil
- 2 russet potatoes
- Kosher salt: half tsp.
- Black pepper, to taste

Instructions

- Let the air fryer preheat to 375 F.
- Wash, and dry the potatoes.
- Pierce the potatoes with a fork all over.
- Coat the pierced potatoes with oil and sprinkle half tsp. of salt.

- Put the potatoes in the air fryer basket.
- Air fry for 40 minutes.
- Take them out and cut them in lengthwise.
- Add butter, black pepper, and salt on top and serve.

3. Mushroom & Brussels Sprouts Pizza

(Ready in about 25 minutes| Serving 4|Difficulty: Medium)

Nutrition per serving: Calories 485|Carbs 58 g| Protein 16 g |Fat 19 g

Ingredients

- 2 tbsp. of olive oil
- 1 lb. of pizza dough
- Fresh thyme: 6 sprigs
- 1 and a half tbsp. of balsamic vinegar
- 4 Brussels sprouts, cut into thin slices
- 1 sliced red onion
- 1/3 cup of grated fontina cheese
- Half cup of shiitake mushrooms, removed stems
- ¼ cup of fresh goat cheese
- Salt & pepper, to taste

Instructions

- Let the air fryer preheat to 400 F.
- On a baking sheet, place the parchment paper.
- Make the pizza dough into a large oval shape.
- Place pizza dough on the parchment paper, and spread a half cup of cheese fontina.
- In a bowl, mix balsamic vinegar with mushrooms. Add onion, Brussels sprouts, salt, pepper, and oil, mix well, and spread over pizza dough.
- Add the rest of the cheese on top and thyme.
- Oil spray the air fryer's basket.
- Bake for 10-12 minutes.
- Serve and enjoy.

4. Blooming Onion

(Ready in about 30 minutes| Serving 2|Difficulty: Medium)

Nutrition per serving: Calories 191 |Carbs 11 g| Protein 3 g |Fat 4 g

Ingredients

For Onion

- Olive oil: 3 tbsp.
- 3 whole eggs
- Breadcrumbs: 1 cup
- Onion powder: 1 tsp.

- Paprika: 2 tsp.
- 1 yellow onion (large)
- Garlic powder: 1 tsp.
- Kosher salt: 1 tsp.

Sauce

- Ketchup: 2 tbsp.
- Dried oregano: 1/4 tsp.
- Horseradish: 1 tsp.
- Mayonnaise: 2/3 cup
- Paprika: half tsp.
- Kosher salt, to taste
- Garlic powder: half tsp.

Instructions

- Cut the stem off of the onion and place it on a flat surface.
- Slice into 12-16 pieces from root down, do not slice all the way.
- Turn and separate the layers.
- In a bowl, mix 1 tbsp. of water with eggs.
- In a separate bowl, mix all spices and breadcrumbs.
- Coat the onion in egg, then dip in breadcrumbs mix, with a spoon coat the onion well.

- Pour oil over breaded onion.
- Put in the air fryer basket and cook for 20-25 minutes at 375 F.
- In a bowl, add all ingredients of the sauce, mix well and serve with blooming onion.

5. Vegan Arancini

(Ready in about 40 minutes| Serving 12|Difficulty: Medium)

Nutrition per serving: Calories 191 |Carbs 11 g| Protein 3 g |Fat 4 g

Ingredients

- Panko breadcrumbs: 1 cup
- Mozzarella, as needed
- Sea salt: 1/4 tsp.
- 2 and a half cups of leftover risotto
- Black pepper: 1/4 tsp.
- Garlic powder: 1/4 tsp.

Instructions

- In a bowl, add breadcrumbs and shredded mozzarella.
- Make risotto into balls.
- Coat the risotto balls into panko mix.
- Keep these breaded balls in the fridge for half an hour.

- Let the air fryer preheat to 450 F.
- Spray the breaded balls with oil and place them in the air fryer basket in one even layer.
- Cook for 8 minutes and serve.

6. Fried Rice

(Ready in about 20 minutes| Serving 8|Difficulty: Medium)

Nutrition per serving: Calories 618 |Carbs 121 g| Protein 14 g |Fat 7 g

Ingredients

- 1/3 cup of coconut aminos
- 3 cups of cooked rice
- 2 eggs whisked
- 1 cup of frozen mixed vegetables
- 1 tbsp. of oil

Instructions

- In a bowl, add cold cooked rice.
- Add vegetable mix.
- Add whisked eggs, oil, and coconut aminos, with rice and vegetables.
- Mix well and place in a dish that is air fryer safe.
- Put it in the air fryer and cook for 15 minutes at 360 F.

- Stir the rice for a minimum of 3 times during 15 minutes.

7. Air Fryer Falafel

(Ready in about 1 hour & 5 minutes| Serving 18|Difficulty: Hard)

Nutrition per serving: Calories 34 |Carbs 6 g| Protein 1 g |Fat 1 g

Ingredients

Falafel

- Flour: half cup
- 1 can of drained chickpeas (15 oz.)
- White onion, chopped: 1 cup
- Parsley leaves: 1 cup
- Lemon juice: 1 tbsp.
- 6 cloves of garlic
- Baking powder: 1 tsp.
- Cumin: 2 tsp.
- Cilantro leaves: half cup
- Salt: 1 tsp.
- Fresh dill leaves: ¼ cup

Instructions

- In a food processor, add all ingredients. Pulse on high until it forms a crumbly mixture.
- Keep scraping the bowl, as required.
- Take out in a bowl and keep in the fridge for one hour.
- With a scooper, take 1 tbsp. of dough and make into falafels.
- Oil spray the air fryer's basket; let the air fryer preheat to 375 F.
- Put falafels in the basket of the air fryer in one even layer.
- Cook at 375 F for 15 minutes.
- Take out and let them cool slightly.
- Serve with tahini sauce and hummus.

8. General Tso's Cauliflower

(Ready in about 45 minutes| Serving 4|Difficulty: Medium)

Nutrition per serving: Calories 246 |Carbs 34 g| Protein 8 g |Fat 6 g

Ingredients

- Cauliflower florets: 6 cups
- All-purpose flour: half cup
- Club soda: 3/4 cup
- Salt: 1 tsp.

- Cornstarch: half cup
- Baking powder: 1 tsp.

Sauce

- Sugar: 3 tbsp.
- 3 minced clove of garlic
- Soy sauce: 3 tbsp.
- Orange juice: 1/4 cup
- Rice vinegar: 2 tbsp.
- Sesame oil: 2 tsp.
- Grated gingerroot: 1 tsp.
- Vegetable broth: 3 tbsp.
- Canola oil: 2 tsp.
- Orange zest: half tsp.
- Cornstarch: 2 tsp.

Instructions

- Let the air fryer preheat to 400 F.
- In a bowl, mix baking powder, flour, salt, and cornstarch.
- Add in soda and mix well; the batter should be thin.
- Coat the florets in the batter and place them on a wire rack. Let them rest for five minutes.
- Oil spray the air fryer's tray. Place florets in the tray and cook for 10 to 12 minutes.

- In a bowl, add all sauce ingredients on medium flame and cook for 2 to 4 minutes.
- Add some crushed chili pepper if you like.
- Coat the cauliflower in sauce and serve with rice.

9. Air Fried Buttermilk Tofu

(Ready in about 2 hours & 35 minutes| Serving 2|Difficulty: Hard)

Ingredients

- Salt: 1 tsp.
- Block of firm tofu (8 oz.) Slice into 4 slices
- Black pepper: half tsp.
- Cornstarch: 1/3 cup
- Salt: 1 tbsp.
- Garlic powder: 1 tbsp.
- All-purpose flour: 1 and a half cups
- Cayenne: 2 tsp.
- Onion powder: 1 tbsp.
- Paprika: 1 tbsp.
- 1 Egg whisked with 1 tbsp. of water
- Hot sauce: 1 tbsp.
- Soymilk: 1 cup mix with two tsp. of apple cider
- Bourbon: 2 tbsp.

Instructions

- Season the tofu slices with salt and pepper, let it rest for one hour.
- In a bowl, add all dry ingredients.
- In another bowl, add all wet ingredients.
- Dip the tofu in dry ingredients and coat in wet ingredients.
- Sprinkle flour mix on wet tofu and pat to adhere.
- Keep in the fridge for half an hour. Oil spray the breaded tofu.
- Air fry them at 400 F for ten minutes, turn the slices halfway through.
- Serve right away with rice.

10. Cheesy Spinach Wontons

(Ready in about 14 minutes| Serving 16-20|Difficulty: Medium)

Nutrition per serving: Calories 281 |Carbs 32 g| Protein 12 g |Fat 12 g

Ingredients

- 1 and a half cups of chopped baby spinach
- Wonton wrappers: 16 to 20
- Softened cream cheese: half cup

- Salt & pepper, to taste

Instructions

- In a bowl, mix spinach with cream cheese.
- Season with salt and black pepper.
- Place wonton wrappers on a flat surface and put 1 teaspoon of spinach mixture in the middle.
- Moisten the edges and make them into a triangle and seal the edges.
- Put in the basket of air fryer in one even layer cook for 6 minutes at 400 F.
- Serve with your favorite dipping sauce.

11. Chili Garlic Tofu

(Ready in about 25 minutes| Serving 5|Difficulty: Medium)

Nutrition per serving: Calories 165 |Carbs 21 g| Protein 7 g |Fat 7 g

Ingredients

- Cornstarch: half cup
- Chili garlic sauce: 2 tbsp.
- Olive oil: 1 tbsp.
- 1 pack of firm tofu
- Soy sauce: 1/4 cup
- 1 and a half tbsp. of brown sugar

- Sesame oil: 1 tsp.
- 2 minced clove of garlic
- Two green onions, cut into slices
- Rice vinegar: 1 tbsp.
- Grated ginger: 1 tsp.
- Sesame seeds, toasted: half tsp.

Instructions

- Press the tofu wrapped in a paper towel by placing a cast iron on it for half an hour.
- Dice the tofu in small cubes.
- Add tofu cubes and cornstarch in a reseal able bag. Shake the tofu and take out in a bowl and pour 1 tbsp. of olive oil all over and toss.
- Cook the tofu in the air fryer for 15 minutes at 370 F., spray with oil more halfway through cooking.
- Take the tofu out in a bowl.
- In a skillet, add garlic, soy sauce, brown sugar, ginger, chili garlic sauce, and vinegar.
- Let it simmer for 60 seconds.
- Add tofu and sesame oil and cook for 60 seconds.
- Top with green onion and seeds, serve.

12. Roasted Green Beans

(Ready in about 35 minutes| Serving 6|Difficulty: Medium)

Nutrition per serving: Calories 76 |Carbs 8 g| Protein 3 g |Fat 5 g

Ingredients

- 1 red onion, cut into thin slices
- 1 pound of fresh green beans, slice in half
- Italian seasoning: 1 tsp.
- Half pound of mushrooms, cut into slices
- Pepper: 1/8 tsp.
- Olive oil: 2 tbsp.
- Salt: 1/4 tsp.

Instructions

- Let the air fryer preheat to 375 F.
- In a bowl, add all ingredients, mix well.
- Oil spray the air fryer's basket and place vegetables in the air fryer basket.
- Cook for 8 to 10 minutes. Shake the basket halfway through cooking.

13. Greek Breadsticks

(Ready in about 35 minutes| Serving 32|Difficulty: Medium)

Nutrition per serving: Calories 76 |Carbs 21 g| Protein 1 g |Fat 5 g

Ingredients

- Parmesan cheese, grated: 2 tbsp.
- Marinated artichoke hearts: 1/4 cup, quartered & drained
- 1 pack of puff pastry (17.3 oz.)
- Greek olives, pitted: 2 tbsp.
- Sesame seeds: 2 tsp.
- 1 can of (6 and a half oz.) artichoke & spinach cream cheese, spreadable
- 1 egg
- Water: 1 tbsp.

Instructions

- Let the air fryer preheat to 325 F.
- In a food processor, add olives, artichoke. Pulse till chopped.
- On a floured surface, place one sheet of dough, add half cream cheese mix on the half of dough.

- Place artichoke mix on top, spread the Parmesan cheese (half), cover the filling with the other half of the dough. Seal the edges.
- Do the process all over with the rest of the ingredients.
- Mix water with egg, and brush the top of the dough.
- Top with sesame seeds.
- Sprinkle with sesame seeds, and slice into 16 strips. Make them twisted strips.
- Oil spray the air fryer's basket and cook them for 12 to 15 minutes.
- Serve with tzatziki sauce

14. Mushroom Roll-Ups

(Ready in about 40 minutes| Serving 10|Difficulty: Medium)

Nutrition per serving: Calories 291|Carbs 31 g| Protein 8 g |Fat 16 g

Ingredients

- 4 oz. of ricotta cheese
- Olive oil: 2 tbsp.
- Dried oregano: 1 tsp.
- Flour tortillas: 10
- Dried thyme: 1 tsp.

- 8 oz. of Portobello mushrooms, chopped without gills
- Red pepper flakes: half tsp.
- 1 pack of softened cream cheese, (8 oz.)
- Salt: 1/4 tsp.

Instructions

- In a pan, sauté mushrooms for four minutes; add salt, thyme, oregano, and pepper flakes. Cook for 4 to 6 more minutes, till browned. Let it cool.
- In a bowl, mix all cheeses and add in the mushroom mix.
- On every tortilla place 3 tbsp. of the mushroom mix on the lower end and roll tightly and secure with toothpicks.
- Let the air fryer preheat to 400 F.
- Oil spray the air fryer's basket and place the tortilla in the basket.
- Cook for 9 to 11 minutes, take toothpicks out, and serve.

15. Charred Cauliflower Tacos

(Ready in about 25 minutes| Serving 4|Difficulty: Medium)

Nutrition per serving: Calories 287|Carbs 19 g| Protein 19 g |Fat 6 g

Ingredients

- Black pepper: 1/4 tsp.

- Avocado oil: 2 tbsp.

- 1 avocado

- Red onion, chopped: 2 tbsp.

- 1 head of cauliflower, cut into florets

- Garlic powder: half tsp.

- Salt: 1/4 tsp.

- Taco seasoning: 2 tsp.

- Corn tortillas: 8

- Lime juice: 2 tsp.

- Purple cabbage, shredded: half cup

- Chopped cilantro: 1/4 cup

- Cooked corn: half cup

Instructions

- Let the air fryer preheat to 390 F.
- In a bowl, mix cauliflower with taco seasoning and avocado oil.
- Oil spray the air fryer's basket generously.
- Put cauliflower in the basket and cook for ten minutes. Keep shaking the basket after every 4 minutes.

- In a bowl, mash the avocado and mix with onion, pepper, cilantro, garlic powder, lime juice, and salt.
- In each tortilla, put 1 tbsp. of avocado sauce and add cabbage, corn, and top with air-fried cauliflower.
- Serve right away.

16. Sesame Tempeh Slaw

(Ready in about 2 hours & 20 minutes| Serving 2|Difficulty: Hard)

Nutrition per serving: Calories 267|Carbs 7 g| Protein 19 g |Fat 6 g

Ingredients

- 8 oz. of tempeh, cut into 1" pieces
- Hot water: 2 cups
- Salt: 1 tsp.
- Rice vinegar: 2 tbsp.
- Cabbage slaw: 4 cups
- Water: 1 tbsp.
- Soy sauce: 2 tbsp.
- Ginger: half tsp.
- Chopped cilantro: 2 tbsp.

- Peanut dressing: 4 tbsp.

- Black pepper: ¼ tsp.

- Sesame oil: 2 tsp.

- 1 minced clove of garlic

- Half jalapeño, thinly sliced

- Chopped peanuts: 2 tbsp.

Instructions

- In a bowl, add salt, hot water, and tempeh. Mix well and let it sit for ten minutes.

- Take tempeh out and drain the water.

- In a bowl, mix jalapeño, sesame oil, soy sauce, pepper, vinegar, garlic, water, and ginger.

- Mix well and pour all over tempeh and cover it, keep in the fridge for 2 hours.

- Let the air fryer preheat to 370 F.

- Take tempeh and discard the rest.

- Oil spray the air fryer's basket and place tempeh inside.

- Cook for four minutes, turn them and cook for four more minutes.

- In a bowl, mix Peanut Dressing with slaw, add peanuts and cilantro, divide into four plates, and top with tempeh and serve.

17. Black Bean Empanadas

(Ready in about 45 minutes| Serving 12|Difficulty: Hard)

Nutrition per serving: Calories 237|Carbs 19 g| Protein 21 g |Fat 5 g

Ingredients

- Salt: 1 tsp.

- Cold unsalted butter: half cup

- Purple cabbage, shredded: 1 cup

- 1 whole egg

- Milk: half cup

- Jack cheese, shredded: 1 cup

- Salsa: 1/4 cup

- One can of black beans (14.5-oz.) Drained & rinsed

- All-purpose flour: 1 and a half cups

- Whole-wheat flour: 1 cup

- Chopped cilantro: 1/4 cup

Instructions

- In a food processor, add butter, all flours, and salt. Pulse for two minutes.

- Add in egg and process for half a minute.

- Add milk while the machine is running, 1 tbsp. at one time, only use enough milk that is required. Make into a dough that will form into a ball.

- Rest the dough at the kitchen counter for half an hour.

- In a bowl, mix cabbage, salsa, cheese, cilantro, and beans.

- Slice the dough in half and make it into 2 balls; make six pieces from every ball, a total of 12 pieces.

- Make every piece into a six" circle and put 4 tbsp. of filling in the middle and fold the other half overfilling. Crimp and seal the edges.

- Make a little slit on top. Repeat with the rest of the filling and dough.

- Let the air fryer preheat to 350 F.

- Place empanadas in the basket of air fryer in one even layer and spray with oil, cook for 3 to 4 minutes.

- Flip and spray with oil and cook for 3 to 4 more minutes

- Serve with Greek yogurt.

18. Roasted Vegetable Pita Pizza

(Ready in about 30 minutes| Serving 4|Difficulty: Medium)

Nutrition per serving: Calories 287|Carbs 20 g| Protein 11 g |Fat 5 g

Ingredients

- Olive oil: 1 tsp.

- Shredded mozzarella cheese: half cup

- Black pepper: 1/8 tsp.

- Pesto sauce: 6 tbsp.

- Salt: 1/8 tsp.

- 1 red bell pepper, slice into quarters without seeds

- 1/4 red onion, cut into thin slices

- Two pita breads (6")

Instructions

- Let the air fryer preheat to 400 F.

- In a bowl, mix the bell peppers with salt, oil, and black pepper.

- Air fry the bell peppers for 15 minutes, shake the basket after every five minutes.

- Take out the peppers. Change the air fryer to 350 F.

- On every pita bread, spread pesto sauce, place vegetables and cheese on top.

- Oil spray the air fryer's basket.

- Place the pita bread in the basket of the air fryer.

- Cook for 5-8 minutes, until cheese has melted.

- Serve right away.

19. Eggplant Parmesan

(Ready in about 40 minutes| Serving 4|Difficulty: Medium)

Nutrition per serving: Calories 189|Carbs 18 g| Protein 5 g |Fat 11 g

Ingredients

- Dried oregano: half tsp.

- Salt: 2 tsp.

- All-purpose flour: half cup

- Dried thyme: 1 tsp.

- 1 round eggplant, cut in half "thick circles

- 2 whole eggs

- Marinara sauce: 2 cups

- Breadcrumbs: 1 cup

- Grated parmesan: 1/4 cup

Instructions

- Put slices of eggplant on a baking sheet and sprinkle with salt (1 and a half tsp.)

- Press the eggplants with a skillet with paper towels on slices. Let it rest like this for half an hour.

- In a bowl, mix salt (1/4 tsp.), flour, and thyme.

- In another bowl, beat the eggs.

- In a separate bowl, mix salt (1/4 tsp.), parmesan cheese (1/4 cup), breadcrumbs, and oregano

- Let the air fryer preheat to 370 degrees.

- Take out the eggplant slices.

- Coat in the flour mix, then in egg, and lastly in the bread crumbs mix.

- Put these coated slices in the basket of air fryer in one even layer and cook for five minutes. Turn them, spray with oil and cook for five more minutes.

- In a pan, add marinara sauce on medium flame.

- Place 1 tsp. of warm marinara over eggplant slices and serve with cheese on top.

20. Seasoned Asparagus

(Ready in about 13 minutes| Serving 4|Difficulty: Easy)

Nutrition per serving: Calories 32|Carbs 0 g| Protein 0 g |Fat 3 g

Ingredients

- Garlic Salt, to taste
- 1 bunch of asparagus

Instructions

- Cut the asparagus off, about 2" from the stem.
- Place the asparagus in the air fryer basket.
- Spray with oil and season with garlic salt.
- Cook for five minutes at 390.
- Shake the basket and cook for five more minutes.

21. Wrapped Corn on the Cob

(Ready in about 13 minutes| Serving 4|Difficulty: Easy)

Nutrition per serving: Calories 207|Carbs 22 g| Protein 11 g |Fat 10 g

Ingredients

- 8 bacon slices
- 4 Corn on the Cob

Instructions

- Put foil piece in the air fryer basket.

- With bacon slices wrap the corns.

- Air fry them for ten minutes at 355 F.

- Serve right away

22. Honey Roasted Carrots

(Ready in about 15 minutes| Serving 4|Difficulty: Easy)

Nutrition per serving: Calories 176|Carbs 2 g| Protein 5 g |Fat 5 g

Ingredients

- Salt & pepper, to taste
- Olive oil: 1 tbsp.
- Baby carrots: 3 cups

- Honey: 1 tbsp.

Instructions

- In a bowl, add all ingredients and toss to coat.
- Place the carrots in the air fryer and cook for 12 to 20 minutes, at 390 F.
- Serve with fresh herbs on top.

23. Avocado Boats

(Ready in about 15 minutes| Serving 4|Difficulty: Medium)

Nutrition per serving: Calories 211|Carbs 9 g| Protein 14 g |Fat 5 g

Ingredients

- 2 avocados, cut in halves
- 4 eggs
- 2 plum tomatoes, diced without seeds
- Fresh cilantro, chopped: 2 tbsp.
- Black pepper: 1/4 tsp.
- Diced red onion: 1/4 cup
- Lime juice: 1 tbsp.
- Salt: half tsp.

Instructions

- Take the pulp out of the avocado, leaving the skin behind.
- Cut the pulp into dices and put in a bowl. Mix with salt, tomato, black pepper, cilantro and onion. Cover and keep in the fridge.
- Let the air fryer preheat to 350 F.
- Place each shell of avocado in the foil to give extra support and place in air fryer.
- In each shell, add an egg and air fry for 5-7 minutes.
- Take them out and serve with salsa.

24. Artichoke Hearts

(Ready in about 15 minutes| Serving 4|Difficulty: Medium)

Ingredients

- 2 to 3 cans of Artichokes, quartered drained
- Salt and black pepper, to taste
- Panko breadcrumbs: 1 cup
- Mayonnaise: half cup
- Grated Parmesan: ⅓ cup

Instructions

- Pat dry the artichokes with paper towels.

- In a bowl, add all of the ingredients, except for bread crumbs, and coat well.

- In a zip lock bag, add bread crumbs and seasoned artichokes and shake well.

- Air fry the artichokes for 10 to 15 minutes at 370 F.

- Serve with parsley and parmesan on top.

25. Garlic Mushrooms

(Ready in about 25 minutes| Serving 2|Difficulty: Medium)

Nutrition per serving: Calories 92|Carbs 4 g| Protein 3 g |Fat 7 g

Ingredients

- Olive oil: 1 to 2 tbsp.
- Chopped parsley: 1 tbsp.
- 1 cup of mushrooms
- Soy sauce: 1 tsp.
- Salt & pepper, to taste
- Garlic powder: half tsp.

Instructions

- Slice the mushrooms in quarters or halves.
- Toss the mushrooms with the rest of the ingredients.

- Put them in the basket of air fryer and cook for 10 to 12 minutes at 380 F.
- Shake the basket after halftime.
- Drizzle lemon juice on top, if desired, and serve.

26. Roasted Broccoli

(Ready in about 25 minutes| Serving 4|Difficulty: Medium)

Nutrition per serving: Calories 70|Carbs 5 g| Protein 2 g |Fat 4 g

Ingredients

- Avocado Oil: 2 tbsp.
- 2 minced cloves of garlic
- Black Pepper: 1/8 tsp.
- 2 Broccoli heads
- Lemon juice: 2 tbsp.
- Sea Salt: half tsp.

Instructions

- Cut the broccoli into small florets.
- In a bowl, add florets and all other ingredients, toss to combine.
- Air fry the broccoli for 20 minutes at 375 F.
- In the last 3 to 5 minutes, switch the temperature to 400 F.

- Drizzle 2 tbsp. of lemon juice on all broccoli and serve.

27. Fried Zucchini & Yellow Squash

(Ready in about 30 minutes| Serving 8|Difficulty: Medium)

Nutrition per serving: Calories 334|Carbs 62 g| Protein 12 g |Fat 4 g

Ingredients

- 1 Zucchini, cut into thin slices
- Bread Crumbs: 2 Cups
- 1 Yellow Squash, cut into thin slices
- All Purpose Flour: 2 Cups
- Salt, to taste
- 2 Eggs whisked
- Buttermilk: 1 Cup

Instructions

- In a bowl, add squash, zucchini, and buttermilk.
- Mix and let it rest for 10 to 15 minutes.
- Place flour, eggs and bread crumbs mixed with a pinch of salt in three different bowls.
- Coat vegetables in the flour, then in eggs, and lastly in the bread crumbs mix.

- Place in the basket of air fryer evenly.

- Cook for five minutes on every side at 390 F.

- Season with salt and serve.

28. Cumin Carrots

(Ready in about 15 minutes| Serving 4|Difficulty: Easy)

Nutrition per serving: Calories 86|Carbs 12 g| Protein 1 g |Fat 4 g

Ingredients

- Pepper: 1/8 tsp.

- Cumin seeds: 2 tsp.

- 1 pound of peeled carrots, cut into sticks

- Coriander seeds: 2 tsp.

- Melted butter: 1 tbsp.

- fresh cilantro chopped

- 2 minced cloves of garlic

- Salt: ¼ tsp.

Instructions

- Let the air fryer preheat to 325 F.

- In a skillet, toast the cumin and coriander seeds for 45 to 60 seconds on medium flame. Let it cool.

- In a spice grinder, grind them well.

- In a bowl, add carrots, salt, oil, garlic, ground spices, and pepper. Toss to combine.
- Oil spray the air fryer's basket and place carrots inside.
- Cook for 12 to 15 minute and top with cilantro and serve.

29. Tomato Stacks

(Ready in about 35 minutes| Serving 8|Difficulty: Medium)

Nutrition per serving: Calories 114|Carbs 18 g| Protein 6 g |Fat 2 g

Ingredients

- Lime zest: ¼ tsp.
- 2 red tomatoes
- Lime juice: 2 tbsp.
- 2 egg whites, whisked
- Chopped fresh thyme: 1 tsp.
- Pepper: half tsp.
- 2 green tomatoes
- Mayonnaise: 1/4 cup
- Salt: ¼ tsp.
- All-purpose flour: 1/4 cup
- 8 bacon slices
- Cornmeal: 3/4 cup

Instructions

- Let the air fryer preheat to 375 F.
- In a bowl, mix thyme, pepper (1/4 tsp.), lime juice, and zest. Keep in the fridge.
- Place flour, egg whites and cornmeal mixed with salt and pepper (1/4 tsp.) in three different bowls.
- Slice each tomato into four slices.
- Coat the slices in flour, then in egg, and lastly in cornmeal.
- Place in the oil sprayed air fryer basket in one even layer, cook for 4 to 6 minutes, flip and spray with oil cook for 4 to 6 more minutes.
- Place tomatoes in stacks in alternate colors and serve.

30. Chickpea Fritters

(Ready in about 25 minutes| Serving 24|Difficulty: Medium)

Nutrition per serving: Calories 34|Carbs 5 g| Protein 1 g |Fat 1 g

Ingredients

- 1 can of (15 oz.) chickpeas, rinsed
- Sugar: 2 tbsp.
- Plain yogurt: 1 cup

- Salt: half tsp.
- Pepper: half tsp.
- Ground ginger: half tsp.
- Honey: 1 tbsp.
- Red pepper flakes: half tsp.
- Ground cumin: 1 tsp.
- Baking soda: half tsp.
- Salt: half tsp.
- 1 egg
- Garlic powder: half tsp.
- 2 green onions, cut into thin slices
- Fresh cilantro: half cup

Instructions

- Let the air fryer preheat to 400 F.
- In a food processor, add seasonings and chickpeas, pulse till finely chopped.
- Add in baking soda, egg, and pulse again.
- Take out in a bowl, add green onions and cilantro.
- In another bowl, add the rest of the ingredients mix, and set it aside.
- Oil spray the air fryer's basket and place tbsp. of chickpea mix on the air fryer tray, and cook for 5 to 6 minutes.

- Serve with prepared sauce and enjoy.

31. Air Fryer Bacon

(Ready in about 10 minutes| Serving 2|Difficulty: Easy)

Ingredients

- 3 to 7 Bacon slices, cut in half

Instructions

- In the basket of the air fryer, place bacon slices in one even layer.
- Cook for nine minutes at 350 F, or until crispy.
- Do not overcook the bacon and serve.

Chapter 8: Air-Fry Dessert Recipes

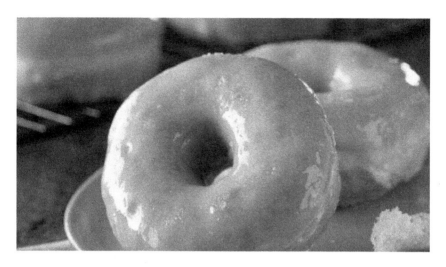

1. Chocolate Chip Oatmeal Cookies

(Ready in about 30 minutes| Serving 6 dozen| Difficulty: Medium)

Nutrition per serving: Calories 102|Carbs 13 g| Protein 2 g |Fat 5 g

Ingredients

- Softened butter: 1 cup
- Semisweet chocolate chips: 2 cups
- Sugar: 3/4 cup
- Packed brown sugar: 3/4 cup
- Quick-cooking oats: 3 cups
- 2 whole eggs at room temperature

- 1 and a half cups all-purpose flour
- Vanilla extract: 1 tsp.
- Baking soda: 1 tsp.
- Chopped nuts: 1 cup
- 1 pack of (3.4 oz.) Vanilla pudding instant mix
- Salt: 1 tsp.

Instructions

- Let the air fryer preheat to 325 F.
- In a mixing bowl, add sugars and butter and cream them for 5 to 7 minutes until fluffy and light. Add in vanilla and eggs.
- In a separate bowl, mix baking soda, oats, salt, dry pudding mix, and flour.
- Carefully add in the cream mix, add in nuts and chocolate chips.
- Place dough on a baking sheet. Divide by tablespoon and flatten it lightly.
- Place cookies in an oiled air fryer basket in one even layer.
- Cook for 8 to 10 minutes.
- Take out and cool them, then serve.

2. Nutella Doughnut Mini Holes

(Ready in about 35 minutes| Serving 32| Difficulty: Medium)

Nutrition per serving: Calories 94|Carbs 10 g| Protein 1 g |Fat 6 g

Ingredients

- Nutella: 2/3 cup
- 1 whole egg
- 1 tube of flaky biscuits, refrigerated (8 biscuits)
- 1 tbsp. water

Instructions

- Let the air fryer preheat to 300 F.
- In a bowl, whisk water with egg.
- On a clean surface, sprinkle some flour, roll every biscuit in a six-inch circle, further slice into four triangles.
- Brush with egg wash. Add one tsp. of Nutella to each triangle.
- Fold the filling in every wedge, seal the edges.
- No need to oil spray the air fryer basket. Place mini doughnuts in the basket in one even layer, cook for 8 to 10 minutes, flip them once.

- Sprinkle confectioners' sugar on top and serve.

3. Chocolate Chip Cookies

(Ready in about 35 minutes| Serving 30| Difficulty: Medium)

Nutrition per serving: Calories 94|Carbs 10 g| Protein 1 g |Fat 6 g

Ingredients

- Unsalted butter: 1 cup
- Granulated sugar: 3/4 cup
- 2 whole eggs
- Chocolate chunks: 2 cups
- Vanilla extract: 1 tbsp.
- Kosher salt: 1 tsp.
- Flaky sea salt, for serving
- Packed dark brown sugar: 3/4 cup
- Chopped walnuts: 3/4 cup
- Baking soda: 1 tsp.
- 2 and 1/3 cups of all-purpose flour

Instructions

- In a stand mixer bowl, add softened butter with the paddle attachment.

- Add packed dark brown sugar and granulated sugar, beat them for 3-4 minutes, on medium speed until fluffy and combined.
- Add salt, eggs, and vanilla extract beat until just well mixed.
- Add all-purpose flour and baking soda in increments, do not over mix it.
- Add chopped nuts and chocolate chunks mix with a spatula.
- Let the air fryer preheat to 350 F.
- Add parchment paper in the air fryer basket, place it so air will keep flowing, and leave some space on the sides.
- Add 2 tbsp. of the dough scoops on the parchment paper, leave some space in between scoops, and flatten them slightly.
- Sprinkle flaky sea salt on scoops—Bake for five minutes.
- Let them cool in the basket for 3-5 minutes.
- Serve right away and enjoy.

4. Air Fryer Donuts

(Ready in about 15 minutes| Serving 8| Difficulty: Medium)

Nutrition per serving: Calories 132|Carbs 14 g| Protein 2 g |Fat 9 g

Ingredients

- 1 can of large flaky biscuits (16.3-oz.)
- Granulated sugar: Half cup
- Melted unsalted butter: 4 tbsp.
- Ground cinnamon: 1 tbsp.

Instructions

- In a bowl, mix cinnamon and sugar. Set it aside.
- Place biscuits separately on a parchment-lined baking sheet and cut one" round holes in the center.
- Oil spray the air fryer's basket.
- Put doughnuts in one even layer leaving one" inch space between, and cook for 5-6 minutes at 350 F, until donuts become golden brown.
- Take donuts on a cookie sheet, and brush with melted butter, coat in the sugar-cinnamon mix.
- Serve right away.

5. Air Fryer Beignets

(Ready in about 48 minutes| Serving 9| Difficulty: Medium)

Nutrition per serving: Calories 186|Carbs 26 g| Protein 4 g |Fat 6.8 g

Ingredients

- Melted unsalted butter: 2 tbsp.
- Plain Greek yogurt: 1 cup
- Vanilla extract: 1 tsp.
- Powdered sugar: half cup
- Granulated sugar: 2 tbsp.
- Self-rising flour: 1 cup

Instructions

- In a bowl, mix vanilla, yogurt, and granulated sugar. Mix well.
- Add in flour and mix until flour is just mixed and it forms a dough.
- On a clean work surface, sprinkle some dough. Knead dough into itself two or three times until combined and smooth.
- Take a 4 by 5" rectangle and place dough inside, and slice into nine pieces.
- Divide the pieces and dust them with light flour. Let it rest for 15 minutes.
- Let the air fryer preheat to 350 F.
- Oil spray the air fryer's basket.

- With melted butter, brush the beignets.
- Place in the air fryer in one even layer. Do not let them touch each other.
- Again brush with melted butter. Cook for 7 minutes, until they look dry and starts to brown.
- Flip them and cook for six more minutes
- Take out on a paper towel and dust with confectioners' sugar.
- Serve warm and enjoy.

6. Fruit Pies

(Ready in about 30 minutes| Serving 12| Difficulty: Medium)

Nutrition per serving: Calories 213|Carbs 21 g| Protein 3 g |Fat 9 g

Ingredients

- Raspberries: 3/4 cup
- 1 and a half tsp. cornstarch with 1 tsp. of water
- Granulated sugar: 1 tbsp.
- Fuji apples: 2, peeled, remove core & slice into ¼" dice
- Ground cinnamon: 1/4 tsp.
- A pinch of kosher salt

- 1 egg yolk with 1 tsp. of water
- Apple juice: 1 tbsp.
- Light brown sugar: 2 tbsp.
- 1 pack of pie crusts (2 rounds)

Instructions

- In a pot, add raspberries, apple juice, apples, salt, sugars, or cinnamon.
- Let it simmer on medium flame, cover it, and turn the heat to low. Cook for 15 minutes, sometimes stir until apple becomes tender but not too soft.
- Add cornstarch to the fruit mix. Increase the heat and cook for 1 to 2 minutes, until it becomes thick. Turn off the heat and let it come to room temperature.
- Meanwhile, take the pie crusts out, and with a 4" cookie cutter, cut the crusts and roll them again. You will get 12 rounds.
- Add 1 tablespoon of fruit filling in the middle of rounds. Brush the edges with water and fold the rounds and seal the edges.
- Crimp the edges with a fork, and make two slits on top of the pie, and brush with egg mixture.
- Sprinkle with sugar.
- Let the air fryer preheat to 320 F.

- Add 5-6 fruit pies to the basket and cook for 15 minutes until pies are light brown.
- Take them out and serve.

7. Angel Food Cake Churro Bites

(Ready in about 10 minutes| Serving 2| Difficulty: Easy)

Nutrition per serving: Calories 171|Carbs 21 g| Protein 4 g |Fat 9 g

Ingredients

For bites

- Granulated sugar: ¼ cup
- Cinnamon: 1 tbsp.
- Half cake loaf of angel food

For dipping sauce

- Milk: 1-2 tsp.
- Softened cream cheese: ¼ cup
- Butter at room temperature: 2 tsp.
- Confectioners' sugar: 2 tbsp.

Instructions

- Slice cake into 1.5 inches of cubes.
- In a bowl, mix sugar and cinnamon. Set it aside.

- Oil spray the air fryer's basket and put the cubes of cake inside the basket.
- Cook for five minutes, at 350 F, until they turn golden brown.
- Take cake cubes out and toss with a sugar-cinnamon mix.
- In a bowl, add butter, cream cheese, milk, and confectioners' sugar. Mix it well.
- Make it the consistency you prefer and serve with cake bites.

8. Honey Cinnamon Roll-ups

(Ready in about 45 minutes| Serving 24| Difficulty: Medium)

Nutrition per serving: Calories 140|Carbs 17 g| Protein 2 g |Fat 8 g

Ingredients

- 12 sheets of phyllo dough
- Toasted ground walnuts: 2 cups
- Ground cinnamon: 2 tsp.
- Honey: half cup
- Melted butter: half cup
- Sugar: 1/4 cup+ half cup

- Lemon juice: 1 tbsp.
- Water: half cup

Instructions

- Let the air fryer preheat to 325 F.
- In a bowl, mix cinnamon, walnuts, and sugar.
- Put one sheet of dough on parchment paper and brush the dough with butter.
- Place the second sheet of dough on top, brush with butter.
- Add ¼ cup of the walnut mix to the sheet. Roll it up tightly; start with the long side.
- Cut into four smaller rolls. Brush these with butter and secure them with toothpicks.
- Keep repeating with walnut mix and phyllo dough.
- Oil spray the air fryer's basket and place rolls inside of the basket.
- Cook for 9 to 11 minutes. Take out the toothpicks and let them cool.
- In a pan, add all ingredients of syrup, mix, and let it boil. Turn the heat to low and let it simmer for five minutes. Let it cool for ten minutes.
- Serve with rolls with syrup.

9. Honeyed Pears in Puff Pastry

(Ready in about 40 minutes| Serving 4| Difficulty: Medium)

Nutrition per serving: Calories 536|Carbs 82 g| Protein 7g |Fat 18 g

Ingredients

- Water: 4 cups
- 1 sheet of puff pastry
- Small pears: 4
- 1 lemon, cut into half
- 3 cinnamon sticks of (3")
- Sugar: 2 cups
- 1 egg, lightly whisked
- 6-8 cloves
- Honey: 1 cup
- 1 vanilla bean

Instructions

- Remove the core from peeled pears, do not remove the stems and cut off the ¼" from the bottom.
- In a pot, add half of lemons, water, cloves, sugar, cinnamon, and honey.

- Cut the vanilla bean in half, remove the seeds, and add the beans to the honey mix.
- Let it come to a boil. Turn the heat low, add pears to the pot, poach them without a lid until tender for 16 to 20 minutes.
- Take pears out without syrup and let them cool for a few minutes.
- Strain the syrup and save one and a half cup of it.
- Let the air fryer preheat to 325 F.
- Roll the puff pastry on a clean, floured surface. Slice into half" strips in width.
- Brush with whisked egg.
- Wrap the pear in pastry dough start at the bottom, use more strips if required.
- Wrap all pears in dough sheets.
- Oil spray the air fryer's basket and place the pears in one even layer in the basket and cook for 12 to 15 minutes, until golden brown.
- Boil the syrup, and simmer for ten minutes.
- Serve pears with syrup drizzled on top.

10. Bread Pudding

(Ready in about 30 minutes| Serving 2| Difficulty: Medium)

Nutrition per serving: Calories 729|Carbs 87 g| Protein 14 g
|Fat 22 g

Ingredients

- Vanilla extract: 1 tsp.
- 2 oz. of chopped semisweet chocolate
- Sugar: 2/3 cup
- 2% milk: half cup
- 4 slices of old bread, cut into cubes (remove the crust)
- Half & half cream: half cup
- 1 egg at room temperature
- Salt: 1/4 tsp.

Instructions

- In a bowl, melt the chocolate in the microwave until smooth, add in cream and set it aside.
- In a bowl, add salt, sugar, egg, and vanilla. Mix and add in the chocolate mix.
- Coat the bread cubes in this chocolate mixture and let it rest for 15 minutes.
- Let the air fryer preheat to 325 F.
- Take two ramekins oil spray them, and add bread cubes to these ramekins.
- Put these ramekins in the basket of the air fryer and cook for 12 to 15 minutes.

- Serve with whipped cream and confectioners' sugar on top.

11. Apple Cider Donuts

(Ready in about 55 minutes| Serving 18| Difficulty: Medium)

Nutrition per serving: Calories 318|Carbs 45 g| Protein 3.5 g |Fat 13 g

Ingredients

- Apple cider: 2 cups
- Packed light brown sugar: half cup
- Baking powder: 2 tsp.
- Ground ginger: 1 tsp.
- Cold unsalted butter: 1 stick
- All-purpose flour: 3 cups
- Ground cinnamon: 1 tsp.
- Cold milk: half cup
- Baking soda: half tsp.
- Kosher salt: half tsp.

For finishing

- Ground cinnamon: 1 tsp.
- Unsalted butter: 8 tbsp.

- All-purpose flour: 1/4 cup
- Granulated sugar: 1 cup

Instructions

- In a pan, add apple cider and let it boil on medium flame.
- Boil for 10-12 minutes till it gets half; if it gets too dry, add a little apple cider.
- Let it cool for half an hour.
- In a bowl, mix light brown sugar, ground ginger, kosher salt, all-purpose flour, baking soda, ground cinnamon, and baking powder mix it well.
- Grate the butter stick in the flour mixture and mix with clean hands to incorporate butter till it resembles pebbles.
- Add boiled (but cooled) apple cider and add cold milk, mix until it forms a dough.
- Place dough on a clean, floured surface. Make the dough into one" of thickness. Keep folding into itself and make into one" of thickness. Do it six times.
- The dough should be springy, make into a rectangle of half" thickness.
- With a donut cutter, cut the donuts. Make 18 donuts of the entire dough and keep them in the fridge.

- Let the air fryer preheat to 375 F.
- In a bowl, melt 8 tbsp. of the butter. Add the rest of the finishing ingredients, except for flour, and mix with a fork.
- Place donuts in the air fryer, cook for 12 minutes, flip halfway through, and leave some space between donuts.
- Coat the donuts in the butter mix and serve warm.

12. Caramelized Bananas

(Ready in about 10 minutes| Serving 2| Difficulty: Easy)

Nutrition per serving: Calories 318|Carbs 45 g| Protein 3.5 g |Fat 13 g

Ingredients

- Coconut sugar: 1 tbsp.
- 2 bananas
- Juice of a ¼ lemon

Instructions

- Clean the bananas but do not peel them; cut them in half length-wise.
- Pour lemon juice over bananas.
- Coat the bananas with coconut sugar.

- Put parchment paper in the air fryer basket and place bananas inside.
- Air fry at 400 F for 6 to 8 minutes.
- Enjoy with toppings, like granola, trail mix, and others.

13. Air Fryer Brownies

(Ready in about 40 minutes| Serving 5| Difficulty: Medium)

Nutrition per serving: Calories 318|Carbs 45 g| Protein 3.5 g |Fat 13 g

Ingredients

- All-purpose flour: ¼ cup
- Butter: half cup
- 2 whole eggs
- Salt: ⅛ tsp.
- Vanilla extract: 2 tsp.
- Chopped walnuts: half cup
- Cocoa powder: ¼ cup
- Brown sugar: 1 cup

Instructions

- Take ramekins and oil spray them.

- In a bowl, add cocoa powder and butter microwave until it melted. Mix well.
- Let it cool, then add vanilla extract and eggs.
- Add in salt, flour, brown sugar, and nuts.
- Pour in the ramekins and cook at 320 F for 20 to 30 minutes, or lightly moist in the center.
- Let them cool and serve.

14. S'mores Crescent Rolls

(Ready in about 25 minutes| Serving 8| Difficulty: Medium)

Nutrition per serving: Calories 191|Carbs 26 g| Protein 3 g |Fat 9 g

Ingredients

- Nutella: 1/4 cup
- Miniature marshmallows: 2/3 cup
- 2 graham crackers, crushed
- 1 tube of crescent rolls (refrigerated)
- Milk chocolate chips: 2 tbsp.

Instructions

- Let the air fryer preheat to 300 F.
- Slice crescent dough into eight triangles.

- Put 1 tsp. of Nutella at the wide side of the triangle. Top with marshmallow and chocolate chips and graham crackers.
- Fold them to make a crescent.
- Oil spray the air fryer's basket and place them in the air fryer basket in one layer.
- Cook for 8 to 10 minutes.
- Serve with warm Nutella.

15. Carrot Coffee Cake

(Ready in about 45 minutes| Serving 6| Difficulty: Medium)

Nutrition per serving: Calories 316|Carbs 46 g| Protein 6 g |Fat 13 g

Ingredients

- Dark brown sugar: 2 tbsp.
- Buttermilk: half cup
- Sugar: 1/3 cup + 2 tbsp.
- 1 egg, whisked at room temperature
- Canola oil: 3 tbsp.
- Shredded carrots: 1 cup
- White whole wheat flour: 1/3 cup
- Grated orange zest: 1 tsp.
- Baking powder: 1 tsp.

- Vanilla extract: 1 tsp.
- All-purpose flour: 2/3 cup
- Toasted chopped walnuts: 1/3 cup
- Baking soda: 1/4 tsp.
- Salt: 1/4 tsp.
- Pumpkin pie spice: 2 tsp.
- Dried cranberries: 1/4 cup

Instructions

- Let the air fryer preheat to 350 F.
- Take an air fryer safe pan and Oil spray it.
- In a bowl, mix orange zest, egg, 1/3 cup of sugar, vanilla, oil, buttermilk, and brown sugar.
- In a separate bowl, mix salt, pumpkin pie (1 tsp.), all flours, baking soda, and baking powder.
- Add into the egg and fold in cranberries and carrots.
- Pour into the cake.
- In a bowl, mix sugar (2 tbsp.), pumpkin spice (1 tsp.), and walnuts.
- Add on top of batter.
- Place in the air fryer. Cook for 35 to 40 minutes and serve.

16. Apple Fritters

(Ready in about 18 minutes| Serving 15| Difficulty: Medium)

Nutrition per serving: Calories 145|Carbs 24 g| Protein 3 g |Fat 4 g

Ingredients

- 2 Honey crisp peeled apples, diced
- 2 tsp. of baking powder
- ¼ cup of butter
- 1 and a half cups of all-purpose flour
- 1 and a half tsp. of ground cinnamon
- Half tsp. of salt
- 1 cup of confectioners' sugar
- 2 eggs, at room temperature
- 1/4 cup of sugar
- 1 tbsp. of lemon juice
- 2/3 cup + 1 tbsp. of milk
- 1 and a half tsp. of vanilla extract

Instructions

- Place parchment paper in the air fryer basket and Oil spray it.
- Let the air fryer preheat to 410 F.

- In a bowl, mix cinnamon, flour, salt, sugar, and baking powder.
- Add 1 tsp. of vanilla extract, milk, lemon juice, and eggs, mix until moistened. Add in apples.
- Put ¼ cup of dough in the basket of air fryer two inches far from each other.
- Oil spray them all. Cook for 5 to 6 minutes, flip and cook for 2 minutes more until golden brown.
- In a pan, melt butter until it starts to become brown. Turn off the heat and cool it slightly.
- Add vanilla extract, milk (1 tbsp.), and confectioners' sugar, mix until smooth.
- Pour over fritters and serve.

17. Banana Bread

(Ready in about 40 minutes| Serving 8| Difficulty: Medium)

Nutrition per serving: Calories 245|Carbs 21 g| Protein 3 g |Fat 7 g

Ingredients

- Salt: ¼ tsp.
- All-purpose flour: ¾ cup
- Sour cream: ¼ cup

- 2 bananas, (ripe)
- Baking soda: ¼ tsp.
- Granulated sugar: half cup
- Vegetable oil: ¼ cup
- Chopped walnuts: half cup
- Vanilla extract: half tsp.
- 1 egg

Instructions

- In a bowl, mix baking soda, flour, and salt.
- Mash bananas in a bowl with a fork.
- Add in egg, oil, vanilla, sugar, and sour cream. Mix well.
- Mix the dry to wet ingredients. Do not over mix.
- Add in walnuts and fold them.
- Take a microwave-safe pan, oil spray it generously and place it inside of air fryer and pour the batter in it.
- Cook for 35 to 37 minutes at 310 F.
- Cool it before serving.

Conclusion

An air fryer is a great appliance that cooks, bakes, or roast foods by hot air circulating at high speed around the food and gives the food a delicious, crispy layer every time without using much oil.

Some say they are just like a convection oven, but they are more compact and do a better job in half the time required by convection ovens. Even if you compare them to other cooking methods, air fryers are much better than any of them. All you have to do is place your food inside the air fryer's basket and give it time, and you will be serving crispy baked food in no time. These are not all the benefits, but air fryers are easily clean and washable and do not clog the arteries.

Using less power than ovens, which saves resources, money, and time. Air fryers come first at reheating the leftovers too. Air fryers are just like a best friend who is ready to eat with you whenever you want, although pre-heating for five minutes is recommended for most models but not a bad deal when you are in a hurry and want something delicious and crispy.

CPSIA information can be obtained
at www.ICGtesting.com
Printed in the USA
BVHW091621030221
599282BV00014B/345